THE
CARDIO-FREE
DIET

THE
CARDIO-
FREE
DIET

Jim Karas

SIMON SPOTLIGHT ENTERTAINMENT

New York London Toronto Sydney

NOTE TO READERS

This publication contains the opinions and ideas of its author. It is intended to provide helpful and informative material on the subjects addressed in the publication. It is sold with the understanding that the author and publisher are not engaged in rendering medical, health, or any other kind of personal or professional services in the book. The reader should consult his or her medical, health, or other competent professional before adopting any of the suggestions in this book or drawing inferences from it.

The author and publisher specifically disclaim all responsibility for any liability, loss, or risk, personal or otherwise, which is incurred as a consequence, directly or indirectly, of the use and application of any of the contents of this book.

S|S|E

SIMON SPOTLIGHT ENTERTAINMENT
An imprint of Simon & Schuster
1230 Avenue of the Americas, New York, New York 10020
Copyright © 2007 by Jim Karas
Exercise photographs by Beth Bischoff
All rights reserved, including the right of reproduction in whole or in part in any form.
SIMON SPOTLIGHT ENTERTAINMENT and related logo are trademarks of
Simon & Schuster, Inc.
Designed by Margaret Gallagher
Manufactured in the United States of America
First Edition 10 9 8 7 6 5 4 3 2 1
Library of Congress Cataloging-in-Publication Data
Karas, Jim.
The cardio-free diet / by Jim Karas.
p. cm.
ISBN-13: 978-1-4169-4913-8
ISBN-10: 1-4169-4913-5
1. Weight loss. I. Title.
RM222.2.K3372 2007
613.2—dc22
2007001914

Illustration on page 20 is courtesy of Marty Bee/focusonhealthyaging.com.

To Olivia and Evan

Contents

Acknowledgments

I would like to thank my team at Jim Karas Personal Training in New York and Chicago. Your dedication, enthusiasm, and professionalism does not go unnoticed. I've asked you to be the best and I see you striving to achieve that goal. I genuinely appreciate all that you do for the firm, for our clients, and for me.

I am very fortunate to have a small group of very close friends, whom I refer to as my "Fantastic Four." Cynthia, David, Jean, and Mike have been incredibly supportive and truly there for me during the good times and the not so good times. Like a car, I need all four wheels to keep me on course and moving in the right direction, and they do so with a combination of love, brains, a much-needed reality check from time to time, and a good dose of humor. These are all things I need on a regular basis and they deliver unselfishly.

And finally, to my kids, Olivia and Evan. I have heard people describe the term "unconditional love," but I never really understood it until you both taught it to me. As you will soon learn, life presents many challenges, but if you can find a safe and happy place to come home to, then it all balances out in the end. I can't even imagine what life would be like without you . . . now go brush your teeth.

Introduction

Are you interested in losing weight, keeping it off, and completely changing your body shape to the astonishment of all your friends? What if I told you this goal is best accomplished without ever stepping on a treadmill or elliptical trainer again?

I know you are skeptical, but let me ask you something: Have you, like millions of Americans, spent hours and hours per week on the treadmill trying to lose weight? What about the elliptical trainer, bike, stair stepper, or VersaClimber? If so, have you dropped any pounds and kept them off? No? Well, what about spinning? Cross-country skiing? Tae Bo? How about those nice long walks in the spring and summer? Did they help keep the pounds off? No, but they sure were pretty, weren't they?

Aerobics class? Stepping? Hiking? Swimming? No.

Snowshoeing? Rowing? Salsa dancing? *Sweatin' to the Oldies?* Oh please, NO!

The reason is both shocking and completely true: Cardiovascular exercise alone won't help you lose the weight and keep it off. "What?" you're probably saying. "I've been told thousands of times that cardiovascular exercise is the *key* to weight loss!" That's what we were all told. But that was simply the wrong advice.

I ask people all the time, "How are you exercising to lose weight?" Most of them answer, "Cardio." I ask them, "Is it working?" They say, "Well, no, but I just need to do it more often and for a longer period of time." If something isn't working, you are going to do *more* of it? You keep doing the same thing over and over again and expect a different result? Albert Einstein had a name for this type of logic: insanity.

Cardio is mindless. You hop on the treadmill, jump on the bike, or step on the elliptical trainer; then you turn on the TV or pop in the earphones of your iPod or flip through the trifecta of required reading (*People*, *Us Weekly*, and *In Touch*), and off you go . . . to nowhere fast. What are you accomplishing? Absolutely nothing, except a Zen-like trance, during which you should meditate on the following mantra:

Mindless Exercise Yields Forgettable Results

For more than twenty years as a weight loss and fitness professional, I have been working with clients one-on-one and have been leading, teaching, and training a team of the best and the brightest personal trainers in New York and Chicago. We've been in the field, identifying cutting-edge research, testing it, and then bringing the best of the best information and instruction to our clients. After twenty years of experience, I am convinced that cardio kills. It kills your weight loss plan, your joints, your immune system, your body composition, your time, and, most of all, your motivation to stay committed to losing weight. But there is one thing that cardio doesn't kill: your appetite. The more cardio you do, the hungrier you get. You burn a few measly calories, then you eat twice as many afterward. The result? Weight gain, and lots of it.

Cardio is the exercise equivalent of channel-surfing. It's mindless and, as you have experienced, result-less for losing weight.

So if cardio kills, what works?

Well, you could ask Diane Sawyer, Hugh Jackman, or Oprah's best pal Gayle King—though it's tough getting their cell phone numbers. I have them because I helped all three get in the best shape of their lives. We did it within their very busy, demanding schedules—and trust me, I know your life is just as hectic.

In the next thirteen chapters, I will explain to you in detail what to do instead of cardio to get in the best shape of your life in only eight weeks. Now, to be perfectly clear, exercise is essential to weight loss. Without it, you are doomed to fail. Don't think you are getting off the hook by going cardio-free. You will exercise, but you will do the right kind of exercise to see and feel amazing results—in an amount of time anyone can commit to. By the end of the eighth week, you won't believe the difference, and neither will your friends! I will also teach you the right way to eat to complement your new exercise program, so you'll have the tools to lose the weight and keep it off, once and for all. When you are finished with this book, you will understand exactly what to do to look the way you've always wanted without ever setting foot on an elliptical trainer or treadmill again! Mind-blowing, isn't it?

THE
CARDIO-
FREE
DIET

CHAPTER 1

Cardio's Reign of Terror

In 1977 Jim Fixx published his first book, The Complete Book of Running. *It sold more than a million copies, and at the time it was the bestselling nonfiction book ever published. With that one book, the whole cardio craze was unleashed. Since then, we have heard hundreds, if not thousands, of doctors, exercise physiologists, and fitness experts go on and on about all the benefits of cardiovascular exercise.*

In 1981 I was living in London and was about to turn twenty-one. Determined to drop some weight (I just couldn't face that milestone birthday feeling so out of shape), I took up running. I was twenty pounds overweight and trying to quit smoking for the fifty-third time, so I used the running to offset the extra calories I feared I would be consuming when a cigarette wasn't in my mouth. I didn't gain any more weight, but I didn't lose any either. For months I was running every day for an hour to an hour and a half, for a total of about ten hours per week, and didn't lose an ounce. If you eat, eat, eat and run, run, run (or perform any form of cardio) as I did, at the end of the day, you won't lose any weight. Learn from my mistake, and don't blow ten hours a week exercising for nothing.

As running became more popular, high-impact aerobics was also hitting the scene. To relieve some stress and try to get rid of the extra pounds (since the running didn't work), I took up high-impact aerobics, still convinced that cardio was the key to weight loss. One Saturday the teacher did not show up for the eight a.m. high-impact aerobics class. About a hundred of us, mostly overweight regulars, stood around for fifteen minutes until I said, "If someone can find a tape, I'll teach." I had the routine memorized, which is never a good thing (as you will soon learn), so up I went to teach the class. Since the teacher didn't show up for the nine o'clock class either, I taught that one as well.

After that class, the manager of the club approached me and asked if I wanted a job as an instructor. I asked what the offer was and he said, "You get four dollars an hour plus a free membership." So began my career as an aerobics instructor.

From that day on, my doomed relationship with cardio was official. Okay, I want to be honest. I am a recovering cardioholic. I have been "clean" for many, many years, and continue to stay as far away from straight cardio as possible, and I'm in the best shape of my life! But for quite a long period of time, I, too, was adamant that cardio was the key to weight loss. Boy, was I ever wrong.

Here is the rest of my history with cardio, which I refer to as the Karas Cardio Rap Sheet:

- **Low-impact aerobics:** Same concept as high-impact, but less jumping, so it wasn't quite as painful on my body, but I still didn't lose any weight.

- **The Step:** Similar to low-impact, but there was a lot of flailing around like a crazy person and almost tripping and falling as I went up and down, up and down a step.

- **The Slide:** It was sort of fun to slide back and forth on a slick surface. I didn't lose any weight, but I did relive childhood memories of sliding on the ice.

- **Spinning:** Spinning really took the cardio world by storm. To this day, spin class is popular among those who still haven't figured out that all that cardio won't get them the results they are looking for. And for the record, spinning is brutal on your body (more on that in Chapter 3).

- **Tae Bo:** I jumped around and repeatedly popped, or hyperextended, my joints, which can lead to major pain and injury. When you box, you are supposed to hit something, not air.

- **Boot Camp:** Since I wasn't in my early twenties and my daily life didn't resemble a war zone, this wasn't a good fit either, nor should it be for any of you.

I believed, like so many people, that working up a "good sweat" equates to a good, effective workout. Basically: *More Sweat = Better Workout.* This is a common misconception. As with everything else in life, we have to learn to work smarter, not harder, to get ahead.

In the past thirty years since the cardio craze has taken off, do you think Americans, on the whole, have lost weight? In 1987 there were 4.4 million treadmill users. By 2000 that number had exploded to forty million users—more than a 900 percent increase. Consumers spend more on treadmills than any other home exercise equipment. Since 1980, the number of overweight Americans has doubled. According to Duke University, "Sixty-three percent of U.S. adults were overweight or obese in 2005, compared to 58 percent in 2001." Given that there are three hundred million Americans, that's an additional fifteen million

Americans who became overweight or obese in just four years.

How can this keep happening?

It keeps happening because Americans continue to listen to the wrong advice. They want to believe that the answer to their problems is as easy as putting one foot in front of the other, but nothing worth accomplishing is *that* easy.

CHAPTER 2

The Body Weight Equation

Some people are shocked to learn that their present body weight is the function of every single calorie they have ever consumed minus every single calorie they have ever expended through metabolism and activity. Your body weight is simply the result of the following equation:

$$\textit{Calories In} - \textit{Calories Out} = \textit{Body Weight}$$

To be more specific:

$$\textit{Calories In (Food)} - \textit{Calories Out (Your Resting Metabolism}$$
$$\textit{and Activity)} = \textit{Your Present Body Weight}$$

We all know what food and activity are, but what is resting metabolism? Your resting metabolic rate is the number of calories that your body requires on a daily basis if you stay in bed all day, doing nothing. Approximately 60 to 70 percent of your daily caloric expenditure goes toward your resting metabolic rate. It includes the functioning of vital organs in your body (such as the heart, lungs, brain, liver, kidneys, and skin), temperature regulation, and—most important to our discussion—your muscles.

For years I have heard people say, "I can't lose weight because I have a bad metabolism." But according to Steve Smith, MD, an associate professor of endocrinology at the Pennington Biomedical Research Center of Louisiana State University, "The variation in resting metabolism is likely to be less than 3 percent. If two equally active thirty-eight-year-old women are both five foot five and weigh 130 pounds, one might have a resting metabolic rate of 1,800 calories and the other 1,854 calories." That's a difference of only 54 calories per day, about half of a medium-size apple. Guess what else? The more you weigh, the higher your basal metabolism. The heavier you are, the more your heart, lungs, liver, and so on have to work because of the additional size. So if you are overweight, realize you have a higher metabolism than you would have if you were lighter.

Gary R. Hunter, PhD, director of the exercise physiology lab and professor at the School of Education at the University of Alabama at Birmingham, says, "Research shows that building and maintaining muscle can speed up metabolism." This research goes on to say that "muscle burns ten to twelve times the calories per pound each day that fat does—you're boosting your metabolism not just during exercise but all day." If muscle burns ten to twelve times the calories per pound that fat does, and most research shows that fat burns 2 to 3 calories per pound per day, then muscle must burn between 20 and 36 calories per pound per day. Tufts University states that strength training has the potential to increase your metabolism by as much as 15 percent. If you go back to our example of a thirty-eight-year-old woman who is five foot five and 130 pounds and burns 1,800 calories a day resting, that 15 percent increase in her metabolism would translate to 270 extra calories burned (that's ten calories fewer than a full-size Snickers bar) each and every day.

Strength training is the key to weight loss because it is the only way to maintain and build lean muscle, which boosts your metabolism. Most women fear it because of the belief that it will make them big and bulky, but quite the contrary: Strength training will actually make you lean and incredibly sexy. Muscle is natural and aesthetically pleasing to the eye, and it is the key to weight loss. If you have this preconceived notion, then please flip to page 36, where I explain why "getting big" is simply not possible for women and should not be a concern.

In order to lose weight, you need to create a caloric deficit, which means you have to take in fewer calories than your body requires for metabolism and daily activity. Here is an example:

$$1,200 \text{ calories (food)} - 1,700 \text{ calories expended}$$
$$\text{(metabolism and activity)} = -500$$

That five-hundred-calorie deficit will force your body to use some of its own stored energy. Another word for stored energy is fat, of which 3,500 calories equals one pound. If you eat 3,500 more calories than your body requires, your body will store those calories as one pound of fat. If you create the caloric deficit of 3,500 calories, you will lose a pound. That's how you lose weight. A lot of other experts would lead you to believe it's more complicated than that, but it's just that simple.

There are four ways to achieve a caloric deficit:

1. **Eat less.**

2. **Increase your activity.**

3. **Elevate your basal metabolic rate.**

4. **All of the above—also known as *The Cardio-Free Diet*.**

Looks pretty simple, doesn't it? But there is a long-term problem with how we have traditionally addressed the first two ways, and it is the reason

Americans haven't been able to keep off the weight—until now. The only effective solution is number four, *The Cardio-Free Diet*, because it incorporates all three ways to lose weight. Here is why any other approach, bar none, will fail:

1. Eat less. The first problem is that we keep buying books and listening to diet doctors (who are often overweight themselves) and experts tell us to count carbs, fat, protein, fiber, or whatever else is being hawked that day, and that you don't have to count calories to lose weight. Guess what? They are all dead wrong. You *must* count calories to succeed at weight loss. Most people don't want to hear this, but it's the simple truth. If you don't count calories, you have no idea what you are consuming on a daily basis. You are shooting in the dark when something so simple as reviewing and understanding the numbers could get you the results you have always been looking for.

The *Journal of the American Dietetic Association* published a report that showed that "85 percent of women who were asked to estimate the number of calories they ate in a day underreported their intake by an average of 600 calories." Do that just half the time and you've just underreported your way to more than thirty additional pounds a year! Startling research by Judith Putnam, a USDA economist, showed that "80 percent of women underestimated their daily food intake by 700 calories." Another study showed that the more overweight we are, the more we underestimate our total calories consumed each day. The *Journal of the American Medical Association* says, "When you see a book cover that touts 'never count calories again,' RUN."

Even if you successfully reduce your calories, you then come to the *big* problem. Your brain is very smart and adaptive. When you go on a restricted-calorie diet, it says to you, "There must not be a readily available source of food. I must be stuck on a deserted island, so I need to slow down your metabolism so that you can live longer on this limited amount of food. To slow it down, I need to get rid of the most metabolically active tissue on your body. Since muscle burns the most calories, we have to cannibalize some muscle so you can exist on fewer calories." By dieting without strength training, you may end up losing some fat, but you will definitely lose muscle as well. Research indicates that it can be anywhere from 40 percent muscle loss and 60 percent fat loss to as high as 50 percent muscle, 50 percent fat. That's a big problem for two reasons.

First, as you diet and lose weight, your body will require fewer calories on a daily basis. If you go from 180 pounds to 150, your body will not require the same number of calories to function at 150 as it did at 180. Your heart, lungs, kidneys, and so on don't have to work as hard, because there is less of you to service. Plus, every daily activity, from getting out of bed to rushing to catch a bus or train to clearing the table, requires fewer calories simply because you are moving around less body weight and you possess less lean muscle tissue.

Second, if you then resume your pre-diet eating pattern, as most people do once they have lost some weight, you will immediately start to gain the weight back. Your "calories in" part of the equation is going up, because you are eating more, and your calories out is going down due to less muscle, which according to the equation causes your body weight to go up. Only now, you are gaining just fat and not muscle—you are in worse shape than when you started! It is this very phenomenon that I believe is the main culprit behind our obesity epidemic. This is the reason yo-yo dieting is well known to wreak havoc on one's metabolism and why so many Americans continually struggle to lose weight and then keep it off.

2. Increase your activity. Everyone thinks activity means cardio. It does burn a few calories, but the operative word is *few*. Here's how cardiovascular exercise works: When you take a step, either on the ground or on any piece of cardio equipment, your large muscles ask for oxygen, which is transported by your blood and pumped by your heart—it is this process that expends calories. When you raise your heart rate, you burn calories at an accelerated rate. The only way to accurately determine the number of calories you have burned during any activity is by your actual heart rate. People are constantly asking me, "What cardio machine or activity burns the most calories?" A machine does not determine how many calories you are burning while performing cardio. Your heart rate determines that number. It doesn't matter whether you are on a treadmill, bike, stair stepper, elliptical trainer, or rowing machine. If your heart rate is 120 beats per minute, you are burning the same number of calories during any activity. Period.

I am always shocked to hear people say, "Oh, I burned eight hundred calories in the past hour" when referring to their cardio workout. Maybe, just maybe, you burned half that, but you had to work really hard for that hour to burn even that many—and that is for a whole hour! Plus, the majority of cardio machines inflate the true number of calories burned, with the elliptical trainer holding the title of cardio's ultimate "Weapon of Mass Distraction." Everyone loves that machine, because when they enter their height, weight, and age, the readout—which is based on a flawed and generic equation—tells them that they have burned hundreds of calories in just minutes. Whoever came up with that idea was brilliant, as elliptical sales have soared in recent years. Great for the elliptical manufacturers, bad for weight loss, because the calories represented on the machine are just not true.

A *Wall Street Journal* article entitled "The Diet That Works" says, "It takes an enormous amount of exercise to burn a meaningful number of calories. A woman who walks thirty minutes a day, six days a week, will burn a paltry 830 calories a week. Theoretically, it would take her more than four weeks to expend the 3,500 calories needed to lose one pound."

A University of Kansas study conducted in 2002 showed that after eighteen months, women who walked thirty minutes a day, three times a week, only lost 2.1 percent of their original weight. For a 160-pound woman, that would mean exercising for eighteen months would produce a weight loss of a little more than three pounds. That same study took another group of women and had them walk for fifteen minutes, twice a day, for the same eighteen-month period. Do you know what they lost? Any guesses? Nothing. Not a single pound.

The American College of Sports Medicine did a sixteen-month study and put overweight college students on treadmills for forty-five minutes a day, five days a week. At the end of the study, the women had gained one pound. You exercise for forty-five minutes a day, five days a week (that's almost four hours a week) for sixteen months, and you *gain* a pound? And these were college-age women. Just think of what those numbers would be for a middle-aged, stressed-out mom of two!

The second bit of bad news about cardio is that as you become more "fit," you burn fewer calories performing the same activity. That occurs because your entire cardiovascular system improves, which is really the point of doing cardio in the first place, and your heart doesn't have to work as hard to transport oxygen during exercise. The improvement is an increase in the heart's stroke volume. Basically, each time the heart beats, it's able to transport more oxygen-rich blood to the working muscles. As a result, your heart becomes more efficient, and fewer heartbeats equals fewer calories burned. Good for your heart, bad for your weight loss goals. The only way to continue to burn the same number of calories once your heart becomes more efficient is to progress the activity. Progressing a cardiovascular program is accomplished through increasing one or more of the following:

• **Frequency:** exercising more often to burn more calories. Downside: loss of time each week.

• **Intensity:** working harder to burn off more calories. Downside: increased risk of injury.

• **Duration:** exercising for a longer period of time to burn off more calories. Downside: loss of time each day.

Do you want to exercise more often, with more intensity, for a longer period of time—just to keep burning the *same number* of calories? Possessing more lean muscle tissue is the way to burn more calories when performing any activity. Let's go back to our thirty-eight-year-old, five-foot-five, 130-pound woman and assume that she is 25 percent body fat. If, through strength training, she changes her body's composition to 20 percent body fat but stays the same weight, then she has successfully lost six and a half pounds of fat and gained the same amount of muscle. In her "new and improved" state, everything she does in terms of activity, from going to the grocery store to taking the stairs to even getting dressed in the morning, will burn more calories. More muscle on the body equals more calories burned when in resting state *and* when performing any activity—as more muscle fibers are recruited and required during each and every activity.

Finally, here is the biggest reason not to rely on cardio to count as an increase in activity for losing weight. According to an article in *Men's Fitness*, "many studies show that aerobic exercise interferes with your body's ability to build muscle. Canadian researchers found that guys who trained six days a week, alternating between strength and endurance workouts (cardio), had impaired strength gains compared with guys who only lifted weights. This, and subsequent studies, showed that although endurance performance improved (when performing cardio and strength-training), gains in muscle strength, power and size actually suffer."

By performing both cardiovascular exercise and strength training concurrently, you are asking your body to adapt both aerobically (cardio) and anaerobically (strength training), which results in different hormonal triggers. When performing high-intensity, steady-state cardiovascular exercise, the body's chemical response is to release cortisol, a catabolic (or muscle-depleting) stress hormone. As your muscle glycogen stores become low, the cortisol starts to mobilize amino acids in the muscle, and fatty acids in body fat, to use for fuel. Increased levels of cortisol break down amino acids in the muscle tissue for energy—chewing up muscle for fuel *and* inhibiting protein synthesis (muscle building), which contradicts the very purpose of exercise in the first place. The word "exercise" should *only* apply to strength training.

Regular cardiovascular exercise also predominantly recruits slow-twitch muscle fibers, which are more efficient in utilizing oxygen than fast-twitch muscle fibers. By continuing to perform high-intensity cardio, your body will adapt by atrophying (shrinking) the fast-twitch muscle fibers in favor of the development of slow-twitch fibers, so your body can become even *more* efficient at utilizing oxygen. Sure, you are becoming more aerobically fit, but at the same time, you're actually diminishing your chances of building the long, lean muscles that will boost your metabolism and help you lose weight.

The introduction of any cardiovascular activity promotes the use of slow-twitch muscles over fast-twitch muscles—and subsequently causes those fast-twitch muscles to atrophy or diminish. This will occur even if you are regularly performing strength training as well. Fast-twitch muscle fibers are essential for developing your body's most aesthetically pleasing composition (shape) in addition to achieving the overall strength that comes with more lean muscle tissue.

The article also says that the worst thing you could ever do for your muscles is to perform a cardiovascular activity for more than thirty minutes. After thirty minutes, you increase the chances that your body will break down your hard-earned muscle for fuel.

How many times have Americans been told to exercise for sixty minutes a day? For what? To burn a few measly calories *and* your most precious bodily tissue, muscle? Do you see how disastrous that advice is and why it is leading us to continue, each and every year, to gain more and more weight?

Increasing activity with strength training instead of cardio, on the other hand, burns calories both during and after the exercise, builds muscle instead of destroying it, and, if done properly, offers heart health as well. Most research indicates that strength training burns between 5 and 10 calories a minute, depending on the size of the muscle group that you are working. That means that you are burning between 150 and 300 calories in a thirty-minute exercise session, which is more than most people burn doing pure cardio for the same amount of time. Not bad, considering that you then get a huge post-metabolic calorie burn as your muscles repair and, most important, you are left with more lean muscle tissue than when you started.

Many people assume strength training is static and cardio is active. My formula for strength training is very active, and the term "interval training" is far more applicable than "pumping iron." You are not sitting and looking around in between each set or exercise like you've seen many "bench heads" in the gym doing. In my program, you finish one set of an exercise, document, drink water, and prepare for the next movement. You keep moving, and that increase in intensity will translate into more calories burned and improved overall cardiovascular performance—about 85 percent of the benefits of cardio alone. A recent study published in the *Journal of the American Medical Association* followed 452 men for twelve years and showed that the reduction in heart disease from weight training was the same as that of walking, running, and rowing. Strength training does not neglect heart health. It can give you heart health *and* increased metabolism at the same time. In this time-crunched world, who can afford to ignore a "two birds with one stone" solution?

3. Elevate your basal metabolic rate. In order to succeed at weight loss, your metabolism must go up, or at the very least stay the same, but never, ever decrease. If you diet without strength training, you will lose fat and muscle. As a result of the muscle loss, your metabolism will go down. If you diet and perform cardiovascular exercise, you will lose fat and possibly even *more* muscle. As a result, your metabolism will go down even farther. If you diet and perform strength training, you will lose *only* fat, increase your muscle, and make your metabolism go up. Sounds to me like the only winning combination. Muscle is preserved and increased *only* through strength training, and the single most important goal of any exercise must be to preserve and increase your body's lean muscle tissue at all costs. If you are not prepared to combine strength training with dieting, don't do anything—dieting alone or dieting with cardio will leave you in worse shape than you started.

If you want to see the results of a muscle-enhanced metabolism, take the "Jim Karas Challenge." Go to your favorite health club or gym and peek into the very *large* cardio room. What do you see? Dozens, possibly hundreds, of overweight individuals toiling away on the treadmills, bikes, elliptical trainers, and stair steppers. They don't look happy, they're not losing weight, and most of them are just using the cardio as an excuse to watch television. I was recently at Club Industry, which is the yearly convention to introduce the latest and greatest new exercise equipment, and virtually every new piece of cardio equipment comes with a built-in TV. Some even have Internet access. Why is our exercise experience resembling more and more our time on the couch? How many of you are only in need of a remote?

Now go to the much smaller strength-training room. It's one-fifth the size of the huge cardio room. What do you see? Maybe a couple of dozen lean, toned, sexy individuals with great posture and a confident aura. It doesn't matter what gym you walk into—I guarantee this is what you will see anywhere in the world. Which room would you rather be in?

CHAPTER 3

Cardio Kills

I said in the introduction that cardio kills your weight loss plan, your joints, your immune system, your body composition, your time, and most of all, your motivation to stay committed to losing weight. But there is one thing that cardio doesn't kill: your appetite. Let's take a moment to review these one by one.

YOUR WEIGHT LOSS PLAN

In the last chapter, we learned how cardio can help you lose a little weight in the short run but truly does nothing when it comes to taking the weight off and keeping it off in the long run. Once you understand that maximizing lean muscle mass is the only lasting weight loss solution, it's obvious why you are better off never stepping on a treadmill, bike, elliptical trainer, or StairMaster again.

YOUR JOINTS

Think about all the injuries you have suffered since you have been doing cardio: shin pain (mine were killing me when I was teaching high-impact aerobics), aching knees, heel or other foot problems (I suffered a stress fracture on top of my right foot from running), a sore lower back from all the pounding on the pavement (yep, got that, too) or from leaning over the bike handles in spinning class, neck and shoulder pain from hanging on to the StairMaster too tightly and juicing the intensity up too much. This is supposed to be helping your body and making you look and feel better? If you're aiming to look like a hobbling humpback with leg warmers and matching knee braces . . . congratulations!

In April 2006 the *New York Times* ran an article entitled "Baby Boomers Stay Active, and So Do Their Doctors." It says that the bodies of today's baby boomers, who are the first generation to embrace cardio as the preferred form of exercise, are breaking down much earlier in life. If you can believe it, sports injuries are the number two reason that boomers visit a doctor's office. Wasn't all this exercise supposed to keep us healthier? I think the number of doctor visits per year is a pretty good measure of just how "healthy" we are, don't you?

Dr. Nicholas A. DiNubile, an orthopedic surgeon, coined the term "boomeritis" because of all the exercise-related injuries he was seeing. He says that "knees, shoulders, hips, and the lower back all have vulnerabilities that surface over time." It is exactly these vulnerable joints that are being used and abused when we perform most cardiovascular exercises. The knees, hips, and lower back are involved in most cardiovascular machines or activities, but the shoulders do come into play during spinning class and on the VersaClimber, rowing machine, stair stepper, NordicTrack, and the elliptical trainer with arms, to name a few.

Intensity must increase for cardio to continue to burn even the same number of calories, because your heart becomes more fit. For most of us, an increase in intensity leads to overuse, and overuse leads to injury, and injury leads to the end of our exercise program. Excessive cardio breaks down the human body at an accelerated rate, which is why boomers are requiring major surgical procedures or treatments for such injuries as the following:

Knees: Damage caused to the tendons, ligaments, and cartilage require numerous trips to the doctor or even surgery. These days, even people in their early fifties require complete knee replacements.

Hips: Pounding on the hips is causing stress, which frequently manifests in the lower back, and complete hip replacements are sometimes necessary. Jane Fonda just had one. Could it have something to do with all those aerobics videos she did a couple of decades ago (which sold millions of copies and, arguably, millions of hip replacements)?

Feet: Stress fractures occur as a result of the repeated pounding, as well as sprained and strained ankles, and plantar fasciitis.

Elbows: Tendinitis—or "Tennis Elbow," as it is more commonly known—occurs when you overuse or improperly use the joint and put stress on the surrounding ligaments and tendons. This happens to many people who insist on hanging on the StairMaster or using arm attachments on cardiovascular machines that don't fit their size and lead them to hyperextend their joints. Be honest, how often do you adjust cardiovascular machines to fit your size? Don't you just hop on and go?

Shoulders: Rotator cuff injuries commonly occur when you perform cardio while holding weights or when excessively pumping the arms of a machine that is not the right fit for you.

Cartilage: Your joints have cushions (cartilage), which is somewhat like a washer is to a nut and bolt. Cartilage provides the cushion. As you pound away on your joints, that washer breaks down and causes pain and inflammation, commonly known as arthritis. Take a look at the following illustration that shows the effects of arthritis on the hip.

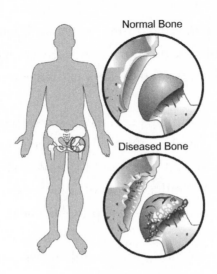

Normal Bone

Diseased Bone

According to a study at the University of Utah School of Medicine, "Overweight and obese adults are much more likely to suffer meniscus cartilage tears in their knee joint." Now, ask these same people, who are carrying an extra twenty, thirty, forty, fifty, or more pounds to perform mindless cardio for hours on end. Then ask them to increase their intensity so they can burn enough calories to actually lose weight. What do you think that will do to their knees? Sounds like a knee replacement just waiting to happen.

For years I used to take my clients out on the beach along Lake Shore Drive in Chicago and give them small hand weights to hold while walking or jogging. That is the worst thing you can possibly do to your shoulders, arms, and neck. I even used them during *high-impact* aerobics classes many years ago. I didn't know any better at the time, and all the "experts" back then said how great they were for weight loss (more bad advice). I just recently saw a class at a health club packed full of people jumping with hand weights onto BOSU Balls, which are an instability tool for strength training and look like fitness balls cut in half. Part of me wanted to race into the class, tackle the instructor, and rescue the students. Do the hand weights help tone your upper body muscles? As I'll explain in Chapter 8, the answer is no. Do they help to increase the number of calories you are expending? The answer to that is yes, but just barely. The increase is negligible, and it comes at a huge cost to your body's joints, ligaments, and tendons.

YOUR IMMUNE SYSTEM

I recently read an eye-popping article in *Men's Health* magazine called "Dying Breaths." In it, author John Bryant talks about the deeply damaging side effects of cardiovascular exercise performed outside around busy streets. When we are sedentary, we breathe in about six to ten liters of air a minute, but when we exercise, that number goes up ten to fifteen times. When you are walking, jogging, or running, you are gulping down "alarming quantities of ozone, carbon monoxide, microscopic particulate matter, sulfur dioxide, nitrogen dioxide, land, and a witch's brew of other pollutants." This can lead to asthma, chronic lung disease, and a whole spectrum of devastating effects on your body.

I experienced this firsthand once with Diane Sawyer, as I frequently picked her up at Times Square Studio after she finished hosting *Good Morning America* around nine thirty a.m. One time we couldn't get a cab to take us uptown, so we walked and jogged from 44th and Broadway to her office at 66th and Columbus in Manhattan (twenty-two city blocks). The next day I asked her, "Did you feel terrible yesterday?" and she, of course, replied, "Yes." So did I. Now I know why. We poisoned ourselves by exercising outside along a busy street—and trust me, we never did that again.

According to Ted Mitchell, MD, any form of moderate exercise can enhance immunity, but "intense exercise actually suppresses the immune-system responses. Studies of marathon runners show a significant increase in respiratory infections at the height of training, indicating that their immune systems aren't functioning at full capacity." Hundreds of doctors have seen the connection between high-endurance cardiovascular activity and a suppressed immune system. Isn't exercise supposed to make us healthier?

An article in the December 7, 2006, *New York Times* entitled "Is Marathoning Too Much of a Good Thing for Your Heart?" reported on a study conducted by Dr. Arthur Siegel and colleagues at Massachusetts General Hospital. The study looked at forty-one men and nineteen women before and after running a marathon. It gave them echocardiograms and tested their blood for troponin, which is a protein found in cardiac muscle cells and is an indication of cardiovascular problems. Before the run, the tests were all normal, but after finishing the race, "60 percent of the group had elevated troponin levels, and 40 percent had levels high enough to indicate the destruction of heart muscle cells." Ponder that the next time you lace up your running shoes for a long run.

YOUR BODY COMPOSITION

Changing your body's composition means an improvement in your lean-mass-to-body-fat ratio. Since cardio does nothing to maintain or build muscle—and could be urging your body to burn muscle—it will leave you with a worse body composition than when you started. Most overweight women possess a body shape similar to a pear, caused by carrying more weight in their lower body, whereby men appear more like apples, because they carry more body fat in the midsection. If women diet or diet and per-form cardio, they may lose a little weight (and muscle) and would there-fore look like smaller pears. Ditto for men—they will look like smaller apples, because they have not built the muscle that would enable them to change their bodies' composition. But your goal should not be a pear or apple of any size. Your goal should be for you to totally change your body's composition in your upper and lower body and your "core" (abs and lower back). That will occur only with strength training. Ready for one more secret? Any interest in great, tight, defined abs? The most effective way to accomplish that visual, inside and out, is to perform strength training for the upper and lower body. I urge you to never perform a standard crunch again. Just like cardio, crunches don't get the job done.

YOUR TIME

- "An hour a day, six days a week!"

- "Four short bursts of fifteen minutes each day!"

- "Do one long twelve-to-fifteen-mile run once a week!"

Do all of these sound as impossible to you as they do to me? In this day and age, who has the time for all this exercise? I know I don't.

In Chapter 8 I am going to show you how to successfully start to exercise to lose weight in only twenty minutes a day, three times a week. Yes, that means in Phase I of your exercise plan, I am asking for only sixty minutes *a week*! That is something we all can fit into our hectic schedules.

YOUR MOTIVATION

In Chapter 6 I talk about being psychologically ready to go Cardio-Free. I know from my own struggle with weight that nothing is more devastating than to attempt a weight loss plan, which includes performing cardio, and fail. You burn though your time, your energy, but most important, your hope. Hold on to a little bit of that remaining hope and let me show you how to permanently lose weight.

WHAT CARDIO DOESN'T KILL: YOUR APPETITE

Remember that every Saturday morning, I used to teach two high-impact aerobic classes a day at a club in the suburbs of Chicago? After class, we would all go to a pancake house and feast. I never really paid attention at the time, but in looking back now, I realize that most of my students were at least twenty to twenty-five pounds overweight. I have come to learn that most people make two mistakes that lead them down cardio's dark path:

1. They believe they are burning thousands and thousands of calories with cardio. Foolishly, they equate the amount of sweat pouring off their head and down their back to the number of calories burned.

2. They rationalize that they can eat whatever they want because, hey, they "worked out"!

If you add up the calories burned from a thirty-minute stroll, they might be 100 to 120—maximum! Many people celebrate that with something like a bagel the size of a hubcap (about six hundred calories). The net effect? You just added 480 to 500 calories to your daily caloric intake. Keep that up for a week, and that's approximately one pound of fat! Keep that up for a year, and you just gained fifty-two pounds and will now have to use the seat-belt extender on your next flight.

Research conducted by Brian Wansink, PhD, showed that people who walked 1.2 miles ate 236 more calories a day than those who didn't walk at all. The reason they ate the additional calories is because their bodies said, "We need more food" because of the activity, or their proud egos said, "Hey, you can eat more—you worked out!" The walk burned around 120 calories, so that created a net result of 116 *more* calories each day for the walkers than for the nonwalkers. What seems like a negligible number of calories can add up to over ten pounds of weight gain a year. To give you another example, I recently gave a speech at Oprah's first live magazine event, called O You!, which was attended by more than five thousand women. I was thrilled to be asked to speak about weight loss, fitness, and improved energy levels. When I asked the audience, "Does cardio make you hungry?" heads started bobbing. I was even a little surprised that they were being so honest, so I asked again, this time louder, "DOES CARDIO MAKE YOU HUNGRY?" to which they enthusiastically responded, "Yes!"

That's what always happened to me, too—I would finish a cardio class or a run, and I would come home starving. I remember standing at the refrigerator with my coat on, because I couldn't take the time to take it off before I stuffed my face. And isn't it funny, it's not just the cardio we do that's mindless, but also most of our eating. We don't even realize how much food we put in our mouths. Remember the phrase *Mindless Exercise Yields Forgettable Results*? The corollary is:

Mindless Eating Leads to Memorable Weight Gain

It's imperative that we stop the cardio *and* the overeating that follows. That's a recipe for failure, but there is another way, which is *The Cardio-Free Diet*.

CHAPTER 4

Turn Back the Clock by Going Cardio-Free

As a boomer, I have every intention of stalling, if not completely reversing, as many of the effects of aging as possible. I'm in the best shape of my life, and I plan on fighting the aging process with a weight in each hand.

After the age of twenty, the average person loses one-half to seven-tenths of a pound of muscle per year. That's five to seven pounds of your body's most precious tissue lost every decade. Some research indicates that by your late twenties, that number could be closer to one percent loss of lean muscle tissue a year. That will make a significant difference in your body's composition and, therefore, your metabolism.

At the onset of menopause, the rate at which a woman loses muscle doubles. So many women have said to me over the years, "What is happening? My clothes don't fit. None of my diet tricks are working. I feel as if my body has taken on a life of its own." They are right! If you continue eating the same number of calories, you will start storing as body fat the extra calories your muscles used to burn. Strength training is the only way to stop the loss of lean muscle tissue. Turn to the next page for a graphic illustration of the loss of lean muscle tissue as you age.

Lean Muscle Tissue Loss—Men

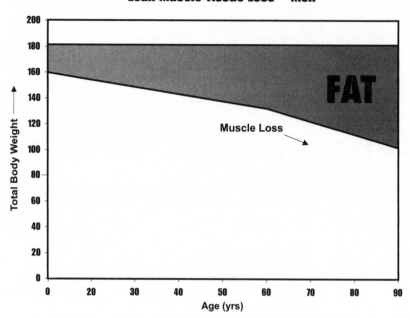

Lean Muscle Tissue Loss—Women

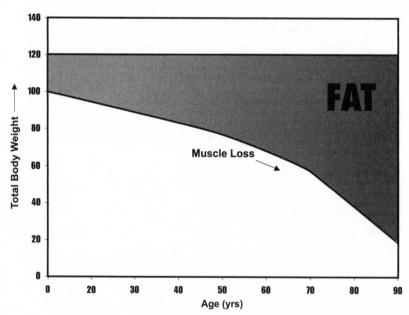

After the age of seventy, the average man and woman lose muscle at the same alarming rate of three pounds a year. So what was a five-to-seven-pound loss of muscle per decade during your "Roaring Twenties" can be as much as a thirty-pound loss in your "Weakening Seventies" if you don't strength train.

For most seniors, muscle loss will determine the difference between living in an independent environment or in a dependent one. I often say in speeches:

If You Don't Lift, You Don't Last

Strength training is the fountain of youth. It's vital to build as much lean muscle tissue as possible and then maintain it *before* your senior status. But even in your nineties, your body has the ability to rebuild your lean muscle tissue. Consider the following results:

• Research from Tufts University showed that individuals in their nineties who strength trained three times a week for eight weeks increased their overall strength by 300 percent!

• A three-year study published in the *Journal of the American Medical Association* found that older and younger healthy men created new muscle proteins at similar rates. Before that study, we believed that the ability to create new muscle would diminish with age.

• Ball State University researchers found that strength training increased an individual's fast-twitch muscle fibers, which are what you use to prevent a slip or fall. Age-related muscle loss, known as sarcopenia, occurs primarily in the fast-twitch muscles. Please note that one-half of all seniors who suffer a fall and break a hip die within a year.

• Researchers at the University of Alabama took a group aged sixty-one to seventy-seven and had them strength train three times a week for six months. The results: On average they lost six pounds of fat, they gained four and a half pounds of muscle, and they increased their metabolism by 12 percent—which translated into 230 more calories burned each and every day from when they started.

It is never, ever too late to start strength training. As a matter of fact, the older you get, the more you stand to gain in overall health from maintaining and increasing your lean muscle tissue:

• increased bone density, which will prevent fractures and breaks

• improved cholesterol levels, which reduces the risk of heart disease

• reduced blood pressure, which lowers the risk of heart attack or stroke

• enhanced glucose metabolism, which helps to prevent type 2 diabetes

• minimized arthritis pain, because when you strengthen your muscles, tendons, and ligaments and you lose weight, you take pressure off of your joints

• diminished lower back pain, as you increase the strength throughout your body (including your core)

• sped-up digestion, which reduces the risk of colon cancer

• lowered stress levels, which are now being identified as the key to a longer, healthier life

• improved golf game. Strength training increases the distance of your drive and the accuracy of your putting, because more strength equals more muscular control. For years this has been my most successful argument with men, who then buy 100 percent into the program.

While traveling throughout the country, I frequently present a speech entitled "The Strength Solution for Seniors" and explain the concept of allostatic load. Allostatic load is a modern-day measure of stress and factors that have been shown to increase or decrease lifespan. These include waist-to-hip ratio, variance in heart rate, blood pressure, blood sugar levels, cholesterol, and, most important, the stress hormones cortisol, norepinephrine, and epinephrine. When you compare this list to the list of benefits strength training offers, you'll see that no one can afford to ignore strength training. In fact, you might be compelled to put this book down and give me twenty push-ups—but I'd be happy if you did just one to start.

The quote "The journey of a thousand miles starts with the first step" applies perfectly to embracing strength training. If you can accomplish one push-up, odds are that in the very near future this number will go to two, then three, and so on, and you will go on to accomplish so much more with your mind and body. I want you to remember this phrase:

Accomplishment Creates Energy

Wouldn't we all like to possess more energy? By embracing strength training, you won't believe what you can accomplish in just a small amount of time.

One final, critical benefit of strength training: Unlike cardio, it requires you to think. With strength training, you have to plan what exercises you are going to perform and concentrate while you are counting repetitions and sets. There is an old weight lifter expression "Link the mind to the muscle," and research proves that the more you simply think about your muscles, the more muscle fiber you will actually recruit during strength training. More muscle fiber recruited translates into more muscular growth. This concentration challenges the brain, and numerous studies prove that the more you expose the brain to new stimuli, the more you keep your brain strong and young.

Walking or any other form of cardio does very, very little to slow the aging process. It doesn't build muscle mass, and it can even accelerate the loss of lean muscle tissue at a time that you desperately need it most. Cardio benefits your heart, but you can achieve 85 percent of those benefits through strength training and get so much more out of the time you allocate to exercise. Any exercise at all is better than none, but if you're going to take the time out of your busy schedule to exercise, shouldn't it be the form that will give you the biggest bang for your buck?

Today very few seniors over the age of seventy-five strength train. Most fear that they will injure themselves or that the exercises will be too complicated. I've taken special care to address those fears in the programs outlined in Chapter 8, as they are safe, effective, and easy to understand.

For many years, my firm in Chicago and New York has provided personal fitness training to clients in their sixties, seventies, eighties, and nineties. You would not believe how a lot of these people look and feel. They have increased overall strength, improved their posture, and eliminated pain, and they walk with the gait and confidence of someone decades younger. Many of them have told me that strength training has changed their lives, and their only regret is they wish they had done it sooner. Two doctors even took the time to call and ask me, "What have you been doing with my patient? I can't believe the difference from their last physical."

In the Cardio-Free Eating Plan, I urge you to cut calories and teach you how to control your caloric intake. Not only will this enable you to effectively lose weight, but it very well may slow the aging process. Researchers from the Washington University School of Medicine in St. Louis examined the effects of calorie restriction on twenty-eight people for more than six years. They found that cutting calories reduced two significant effects of aging, a thyroid hormone called triiodothyronine, which has been shown to help control cellular metabolism and energy balance in the body, and an inflammatory molecule called tumor necrosis factor alpha. This combined reduction slows down the aging process in humans. The results reinforced an earlier study on rats that showed that those rats on calorie-restricted diets lived longer.

By strength training and reducing your caloric intake, you will lose weight, look and feel so much better, *and* add years to your life. How can you even consider any other option?

Your body naturally wants its muscle back. It wants to feel young again, to be strong, to be pain- and injury-free. It wants to bound up a flight of stairs and get on the ground and play with the kids. Challenge your muscles and your brain with strength training, and both will thank you with enhanced performance. You'll lose weight, turn back the clock, and get in amazing shape, regardless of your age.

CHAPTER 5

Cardio-Free Works for Both Men and Women

Most women struggle with weight more than most men. Part of the issue is size (heavier and taller people have higher metabolisms and can therefore consume more calories), but the other significant issue is that women possess less lean muscle tissue than men. Here are a few points to help you understand the difference between men and women and weight loss.

1. Men require only 3 percent essential body fat to properly function. Women require 12 percent essential body fat, because of their breasts and reproductive organs. Women are always going to possess more body fat than men.

2. The majority of women have biological children, which causes them to gain and then try to lose the weight postpartum (which could result in a loss of both fat and muscle). Being a fitness professional for as long as I have, I must say that I am frequently upset by the amount of weight most women gain while pregnant. It is generally believed that twenty-five to thirty-five pounds is totally acceptable, yet I know of hundreds of women who have gained fifty, sixty, seventy, or more pounds during their pregnancies, and their doctors didn't address the weight issue before they ballooned in size. It leaves them with an overwhelming weight loss job when the pregnancy is over.

3. All women go through menopause, which doubles the loss of lean muscle tissue, lowers metabolism, and creates a higher hurdle to losing weight.

4. Women diet more. At any given time, 44 percent of all women and 29 percent of all American men are on a diet. All that dieting, mostly done without the benefits of strength training, cannibalizes lean muscle tissue. Plus, if women are exercising in addition to dieting, they are probably doing cardio, which only compounds the problem.

5. Women fear strength training. I touched upon this earlier, as I *know* that fear of "getting big" lurks in the back of women's minds. That is why only 17.5 percent of women perform regular strength training. In my experience, even those women who do perform strength training aren't using heavy enough weights to achieve real benefits and results.

In twenty years as a weight loss and fitness professional, I have *never* had a female client get bulky from strength training. It just doesn't happen, because women do not possess the natural levels of testosterone that are required to build big, bulky muscles. Some women feel that they are already too muscular, when the reality is that they are simply carrying around a considerable amount of body fat. Body fat is stored in obvious places such as your hips, glutes, and arms, but there is also fat that is stored intramuscularly, which means that the fat is stored within your muscles. It's very similar to a marbleized cut of meat at a steak house. If you have ever looked at a raw steak, you've seen the lines of white fat alongside the red meat. This same phenomenon occurs in your body. You may be carrying a great deal of fat within your muscles, but you perceive that it is just muscle. If only that were the case.

When women lose body fat on *The Cardio-Free Diet*, their muscles will appear smaller because they have lost the intramuscular fat and gained some much-needed, calorie-burning lean muscle. This is the secret of "toning" the body and why you get smaller by strength training.

Those freaky women in muscle-building magazines are almost all on steroids or consuming massive amounts of calories to support that type of muscle growth. That is why they are big and frightening, not because of the strength training. Strength training actually helps women shrink.

When I helped Diane Sawyer lose twenty-five pounds and get into the best shape of her life, she was hitting the strength training hard. She could not believe how her body just shrank. Her arms (she lost close to four inches on each one) were amazing, and, as it was springtime, she made sure there were lots of sleeveless dresses and tops in her closet. Her lower body completely changed shape. Her old skirts were falling off, so she was holding them up in the back with clips and pins on *Good Morning America*.

Ladies, the same can happen to you. You can get incredibly lean and toned, see your whole body's composition change before your eyes, and look incredible. The biggest problem you'll have is explaining your secret over and over again to all your friends, family, and coworkers as they gush over how fabulous you look. Diane was fifty-six at the time, and her body responded immediately. Your body will respond to strength training at *any* age.

After featuring a big story on Diane's success with my program in April 2002, *O, The Oprah Magazine* placed four women, one each in their twenties, thirties, forties, and fifties, on my eating and exercise plan and did a follow-up story in October 2002.

Gayle King, editor-at-large at *O* and Oprah's best pal, agreed to be the woman in her forties. She lost twenty pounds, but the real shocker was the inches lost all over her body, which, like Diane, resulted in gorgeous arms and a drastic reduction in her hips and waist. Look at these numbers:

	Before	After	Loss in Inches
Chest	39.75	37	2.75
Waist	33	27.5	5.5
Hips	44.5	40.75	3.75

Gayle had a whole new body composition (much more like an hourglass), and to this day, she has kept the majority of the weight *and* inches off. Jane Brody, a health writer for the *New York Times*, sums it up best: "Strength training leads to a smaller, tighter physique." She's right.

A couple of years ago, *Sports Illustrated* swimsuit edition cover model Petra Nemcova and I did a television show for the Discovery Health Channel called *Secrets of Superstar Fitness*. I met her in a huge suite at a hotel on Central Park South in New York. Every manager, assistant manager, room service waiter, bellhop, and just about every other male member of the hotel staff had to come up to see if Petra needed anything, and she was gracious and charming to each and every one of them. When it was time to start the exercise portion of the program in the living room, I pulled my SPRI exercise equipment out of my gym bag for the workout. Petra had a huge smile on her face. She quickly went into her bedroom and came out with her own set of the same SPRI Xertubes and Lex Loops, which are used in my first exercise program (pictured on page 63 and 64). Petra says she never travels without them and uses them all the time at home.

Petra is lean and toned, her posture is impeccable, and she has possibly the best body I have ever seen. Muscle on women is sexy. Strength training helps make you lean, toned, *and* strong. That comes in handy when lugging around kids, groceries, purses, briefcases, luggage, or the haul from a major sale at Target. Men, on the other hand, will grow bigger muscles through strength training because of their body's natural muscle-building potential.

In the summer of 2005, I spent eight weeks with Hugh Jackman in Marrakech, Morocco, and London to get him physically prepared for *X-Men: The Last Stand*. Now, keep in mind—this is Hugh Jackman, a man universally known for looking great—and even he admits that he was in the best shape of his life when he started filming, which is a wonderful testament to the program and the work we did together.

The results he experienced were from *only* performing strength training. Men, if you want to look like Hugh Jackman, I strongly urge you to rethink that cardiovascular exercise program.

During the eight weeks we were training, I also did an intense program with his very pretty wife, Deborra-Lee Furness, who is also an actor. Hugh beefed up, but Deborra-Lee slimmed down. On my program, Deborra-Lee got to her lowest adult weight, totally changed her body composition, and to this day looks amazing! She just shrank, especially in her midsection. They both did the same form of exercise, but with two very different effects on the body.

Diane, Gayle, Hugh, and Deborra-Lee were all basically on very similar exercise programs. Most trainers believe that you should work with men one way and women another. That is totally untrue, because the goal for both men and women is to build as much lean muscle tissue as possible. Men have twenty to thirty times the muscle-building potential as women, so why would you ever give a woman a light weight and encourage her to perform dozens of repetitions so that she will "tone without getting big"? Getting big is not possible for her, and that toned look that almost all women desire comes from *building* long, lean muscles and burning off the body fat inside or on top of them. The optimal way to achieve that visual is to perform *only* strength training.

CHAPTER 6

Are You Mentally Prepared to Go Cardio-Free?

Losing weight for the long run requires that you make some significant changes in your lifestyle. The concept of losing weight is simple in its method—eat less, exercise more—but far from easy in its implementation. As most of us know all too well, it's far easier to change our attitudes than it is to change our behaviors.

This is why so many of us are quick to discount the benefits of losing weight or to point out just how impossible the feat is for us. Fearing our eventual failure, we create excuses, which ultimately only serve to ensure our defeat before we even begin. In this chapter I am going to walk you through how to make these simple changes *easier* to implement in your life. This will ensure your success even before you pick up your first weight.

There are four important stages that you will go through before making a change. They are:

- **Contemplation**

- **Preparation**

- **Action**

- **Maintenance**

CONTEMPLATION

For those of you who do exercise already, chances are that frequenting the cardio room at the club or doing cardio outside feels far more comfortable and safe than venturing into the weight room or attempting an unfamiliar strength-training program at home. But you have to step back for a moment and ask yourself, did all the cardio help me lose weight? Are my family members, friends, and coworkers losing weight with cardio? Chances are that no one you know has successfully lost weight and kept it off by dieting alone or by dieting and performing cardio. Let your motivation be that you are going to be the first one to actually succeed at weight loss and, consequently, change your life forever. Who knows, you might even spark some inspiration in others along the way. I'd like you to get out a piece of paper and answer the following questions:

1. Why am I overweight?

2. What is my real motivation for losing weight?

3. Did dieting alone help me lose weight and keep it off?

4. Did dieting and performing cardio help me lose weight and keep it off?

5. Have I *ever* really succeeded at losing weight and keeping it off?

6. Have I ever tried strength training as outlined in Chapters 7 and 8?

7. Have I ever counted calories?

8. What have I got to lose by going Cardio-Free?

Keep that piece of paper in the top drawer of your desk, in your day planner, or in the zipper pocket of your purse, briefcase, or gym bag, as we are going to revisit it later on in this plan.

PREPARATION

If you have decided that you will embrace this program, then you enter the phase of preparation, as you must now get ready to make concrete decisions, such as:

1. What is your start date? Pick a date that makes sense, but don't put it off more than a week. If you wait too long, the urge will pass. Most of us have let that happen in the past, so don't let it be the case this time. In my experience, Monday is the best day to start the program. Monday is a clean slate and gives people the feeling of possibility and new beginnings.

2. Decide when you will shop for the week 1 eating plan. Back into that decision by picking a day and time right before your start date, and stick to it. If you are starting on a Monday, resolve to go shopping on Saturday or Sunday. Don't forget to bring the shopping list on page 212.

3. Determine which exercise program suits you best, and figure out if you have to purchase any exercise equipment. Where will you work out, at home or in a gym? Do you have travel plans, and if so, will you need portable equipment? If you are going to purchase either free weights or the SPRI exercise tubing, go ahead and anticipate that you will progress quickly, which I will explain in Chapter 9. If you purchase free weights, buy five-, eight-, ten-, twelve-, fifteen-, and twenty-pound dumbbells to start. SPRI Products offers an excellent thirty-pound adjustable briefcase. In one small case, you can create up to two fifteen-pound dumbbells or one thirty-pound dumbbell, which is what you will soon need. Are you shocked by that last sentence? Don't be—you will be lifting those heavier weights in no time. Same goes for the SPRI exercise tubing. Buy the green, red, blue, and purple Xertubes and the green and red Lex Loops. That way, you will be ready when you achieve results and need to move your exercise program to the next level—it will happen quickly! You will also save the time it will take to go back to the store or the cost of the shipping if you order it. Don't let those become excuses down the road for not continuing to progress.

4. Where will you perform each session? You basically have three choices: home, office, or exercise facility. At home, find a private place inside to go through the twenty-minute routine, or, weather permitting, you can easily go outside and perform your workout. SPRI Products even has equipment specifically meant to be used outside. Surprisingly, the office is actually a good option. I know a number of people who close their doors and perform the strength training in their offices during lunch. No boss is going to get angry with you for getting in better physical and mental shape, which will only serve to improve your job performance.

5. When will you perform each session? I find that most people struggle with this decision the most. I realize you don't *want* to exercise, but I hope you also realize by now that you *have* to do it. Time is short, so why not get the exercise done rather than talk and drink coffee? In Chicago, I know of a number of soccer moms who exercise while the kids are at lessons or practice. In Phase I of this plan, you need to set aside only twenty minutes of exercise, three times a week. That's a total of one hour a week. Research indicates that those who exercise first thing in the morning are more consistent than those who wait until later in the day, simply because emergencies or last-minute distractions can derail your plans. And let's be honest, when pressed for time, exercise will be the first thing to go. But with a little advance planning, you can make it happen any time, day or night. If your weekdays are too full, I even offer the option of exercising on both Saturday and Sunday and choosing only one weekday to complete three sessions. The key is getting started, so figure out what will work for you. Plus, you can always change your mind. You may think that you will get home from work and exercise, only to find that it preys on your mind all day long. Though you might not be a morning person by nature, you might decide that getting it over with first thing is a more realistic option. Just make sure it happens.

ACTION

As you now enter the action stage, you are going to meet with some resistance. Your "I hate exercise" pals *and* your cardio pals are going to be shocked when you tell them that you are only performing strength training. If you have some walking buddies or friends you used to do the treadmill with at the club, schedule a cup of coffee with them and explain that you are giving something else a try.

It is critical in the action phase that you tell your friends, family members, and coworkers that you are determined to lose weight. Be open and honest about your desire to lead a healthier life. When people don't "go public" that they are trying to lose weight, it's usually because they privately expect to fail before they even get started. You should plan to succeed, and the more you tell people that you are taking positive steps to eat better and perform the right kind of exercise, the more you reinforce that this is not going to be another swing and a miss.

During the action phase, your body will respond to the strength training—your body composition and posture will change quickly. Your body wants its muscle back, and it will thank you very quickly by responding with fabulous results. Whereas most people focus only on the scale when losing weight, you need to keep looking at all the positive changes occurring in your body's composition. The moment you put something on, you will see what I mean. You will get positive feedback from friends, family members, and coworkers, which will give you the confidence and conviction to stay with this plan for good.

In the first two weeks, the number on the scale can drop significantly. That comes as a result of both losing body fat on the Phase I eating plan and losing some water weight. The glycogen stored in your body is a combination of sugar and water. When you diet, that stored glycogen is going to be the first fuel the body uses to make up for your caloric deficit. As you burn though that glycogen, the loss of water will cause the number on the scale to go down precipitously. In the first two weeks, it would be possible to lose as much as eight to ten pounds, depending on your starting condition.

After Phase I, women should aim for one to two pounds of weight loss a week and men should shoot for two to three, depending on how overweight they were to begin with. After establishing their starting weights, both men and women can keep losing at that clip until they hit their goal weights.

MAINTENANCE

Now, there is very little difference between the action and maintenance phases. Once you reach your weight loss and body composition goals, you will find that you must continue to do *exactly* the same things you've done to lose weight in the first place to keep the weight off for good. Millions of people begin an eating and exercise plan with a set weight in mind, but once they achieve that goal (which very few do), they believe they are entitled to go back to their previous eating and exercise habits. That will only lead them to gain all the weight back, and remember, unless they are strength training, that weight gain will only be fat.

When you embrace *The Cardio-Free Diet*, it is a life decision, not a short-term answer. You *are* going to slip up from time to time. Across the board, research shows that if you go on a weight loss plan and think that you are never going to slip up, you are doomed to fail. We all make mistakes from time to time. I know I do, and the majority of my most successful clients do as well. If you had a big celebration dinner or went to a great party with terrific food, then get up the next morning, eat the right breakfast, get in your exercise, and get right back on plan. You might come home one night after a frustrating day and find yourself plowing through a bag of chips. If so, forget about it. Don't adopt an "I blew it" position and just give up. Keep your eye on the long-term goal, not the short-term bump in the road.

CHAPTER 7

Strength Training 101

There are three stages of effective strength training. Let me use a classic bicep curl as an example.

Stage 1: Working Repetitions

When you begin a strength training exercise with either free weights, an SPRI exercise tube, or a strength-training machine, as soon as you curl your fist upward, you are placing some force against your bicep muscle. The first stage of any strength training exercise is called working repetitions.

During working repetitions, you've just started the movement, and it doesn't feel very hard. You are maintaining good form and slowly working a full range of motion, which means fully contracting the muscle on the way up and slowly lowering it all the way down. Always work the full range of motion, as that is what produces long, lean, calorie-burning muscles. Your working repetitions should make up five to six repetitions of a ten-rep set.

NOTE: If you are approaching the eighth, ninth, or tenth rep and you are still comfortable in working repetitions, then the weight/tension is too light. This is the most common mistake and the reason most people—especially women—miss out on all the benefits of the strength training.

Stage 2: Fatigue

Then, when you start to feel the muscle straining and each repetition is getting harder, you begin to enter stage two, fatigue. Your bicep muscle is getting tired. You may feel the need to cheat a little, but you fight to maintain good form, which you should always strive to achieve. The fatigue stage should last three to four repetitions, or reps six or seven to eight or nine of a ten-rep set.

Stage 3: Failure

Suddenly you can no longer move the weight, band, or machine. You just hit the final and most important stage: failure. When you hit muscular failure, you are no longer physically capable of performing even one more rep. This should happen on rep nine or ten of a planned ten-rep set.

Failure is a concept that most people understand, but very few actually implement in their workouts. This is a shame because without it, you are truly wasting your time. I want you to always apply this phrase to your strength-training exercise program:

You Succeed When You Fail

When you hit failure, you produce tiny tears in your muscles. Don't be frightened by that thought. Creating little tears is a good thing, because, over the next twenty-four to forty-eight hours, the bicep muscle is going to repair those tears. But before starting the repair process, the brain says to the bicep muscle, "Hey, the next time you are asked to perform that bicep curl, I want you to get better at it. So, when you are down there repairing the little tears, go ahead and add just a little more lean muscle tissue so that you don't fail next time." Failure during strength training is the only thing that builds lean muscle tissue. Soon thereafter, you will have to increase the resistance so that you continue to fail, which is called *progression*.

With cardio, we never, ever hit muscular failure. Your muscles may get tired, but they are never pushed to the point where they are required to grow, and you never get the benefit of maintaining and building lean muscle tissue. The same thing happens when we stick with five-pound weights and never even attempt failure or progression. If you've had the same dusty set of five- and eight-pound dumbbells since the Reagan era, you know what I'm talking about. You don't start at a heavy weight, as that would lead to a potential injury. You should start out with a comfortable weight and then build up over time. I will help you better understand the concept of progression in Chapter 9.

STRENGTH TRAINING FAQ

Here are some of the most frequently asked questions about effective strength training.

How many reps should I perform of each exercise?

Most people use too light of a weight/tension and perform far too many reps. To optimally build long, lean muscles, you should never perform more than ten reps with proper form at full range of motion. If you aren't hitting failure by the tenth rep, then the weight/tension is too light. You should increase by the smallest possible increment until you find a weight/tension that challenges you to hit failure on or before the tenth rep, without compromising your form or risking injury.

How many sets of each exercise should I perform?

That depends at what level you are starting. As a true beginner, one set (to failure) is all that you need to effectively build long, lean muscles (which is what you will do in Phase I of this plan). As you strength train consistently for two weeks and get more comfortable, I will ask you to go to two sets for one-half of the exercises in the program. You may either perform two sets in a row, one right after the other, or you may perform your entire series of exercises, then repeat to do the second set. Both styles get the job done effectively. As you progress to a more advanced strength and resistance program, you should be performing three sets of the exercises, but this will not be required in the eight-week plan.

What is the optimal speed for each repetition?

Ideally, a rep should take two counts on the way up and four counts on the way down. Using our original example of a bicep curl, that means counting "one, one thousand, two, one thousand," as you curl the weight up, and four such counts on the way down. Researchers have found that eccentric training causes more microtrauma (which is the scientific term for tiny tears) to the muscle than concentric training, and it therefore more efficiently promotes muscle growth. The concentric part occurs as you contract (shorten) the muscle (curl up the bicep), and the eccentric part occurs as you lengthen it back out to starting position. Because you want to stress the muscle more on the movement that will get you better results, a slow two-count is perfect for the contraction, but you want to take twice as much time to lower the weight back to the starting position.

Can I perform strength training every day?

Yes, but you have to alternate body parts, because it takes twenty-four to forty-eight hours for a muscle to repair itself after strength training. If you plan to exercise on Monday, Wednesday, and Friday, the best strategy is to do total body training all three days. You will have Tuesday, Thursday, and the weekend to repair and build the muscles. If very busy weekdays require you to do strength training on Saturday and Sunday, then you should work your upper body on one day (do two sets of each exercise, since you are cutting the number of exercises in half) and the lower body on the other. Your third workout should be on Tuesday, Wednesday, or Thursday, and it should work the total body. An exception to this rule is your "core"—abdominals, obliques, and lower back. Because of the relatively small amount of muscle fiber in each, they can be worked every day.

Make sure you always take off one day a week. My program is only three days a week, but I know that some people get into an exercise program and give it all they've got right from the very start. While this type of motivation is great, it's very important to make sure you take one complete day off each and every week. This enables your body to repair, and you will jump back into your program stronger than ever after the rest.

NOTE: Young men frequently go after their strength-training program so aggressively that they overtrain and minimize the benefits of the exercise. Proper recovery and repair of the muscle are vital to achieving the best results.

Since I had been doing cardio for my lower body, can't I just do strength training on my upper body?

No—cardio never really developed your lean muscle tissue in your lower body, and it may even have depleted it. I find that most women want to train only their lower body, while men want to train only their upper-body "beach" muscles. But you want to train *all* your muscles to maximize your whole body's lean muscle tissue. What's more, *Men's Health* reports that Norwegian researchers have found that beginning lifters gain upper-body strength by doing lower-body exercises. When you strength train and place resistance against your muscles, you trigger a release of hormones, which will stimulate muscle growth throughout your body. Since your lower body uses the largest muscles, they release more muscle-building hormone, benefiting the entire body.

Should I feel sore after my workouts?

When beginners start an exercise program, they frequently complain of what's known as delayed-onset soreness. Most researchers do not know why some people experience more soreness than others, and the whole science of soreness is a bit of a mystery. But if you are not sore, it does not mean your strength-training program has been ineffective. If your body weight and composition are changing, you are getting the job done. Let the scale and your clothes be your guides.

> **NOTE:** "Good" soreness is "Oh, I worked my triceps yesterday, and when I squeeze them today, I can feel that they were worked." "Bad" soreness is "I did some squats yesterday and my knee is bothering me." Please, always be aware of which soreness you are experiencing, and if it is of the bad variety, see your doctor.

If I stop strength training, will my muscle turn to fat?

Muscle and fat are two totally different tissues in your body, with completely different purposes and therefore independent functionality. If, for whatever reason, you ceased strength training (which I hope never happens), then you will lose some of the muscle you have increased and preserved, and that will lead to a diminished metabolism. If you continue to consume approximately the same number of calories, the extra calories that you used to burn up to maintain your muscle will now not be burned up. They will be stored as fat. So the muscle does not actually turn *into* fat, but the reduction in your lean muscle tissue will lead you to a lower metabolism and result in you carrying more body fat.

I used to be in much better shape. Will that help when I go on the Cardio-Free exercise plan?

If you performed strength training in the past, or held a job that required you to lift and carry heavy things, your body, at one time, possessed more lean muscle tissue. When you begin the Cardio-Free exercise plan, your body will remember what you are telling it to do, and you will increase your lean muscle tissue faster than a true beginner. They call this muscle memory. But true beginners, don't let this fact discourage you. You too will see drastic changes in your body in a very short period of time.

I find that I hold my breath when performing strength training. What is the optimal way to breathe?

There is a general rule that works very effectively: Exhale on the contraction, or exertion, and inhale when returning to the starting position. Please make sure never to hold your breath. Breathe slowly, as if you are sipping the air in and blowing it out through a straw. When you breathe in slowly, you optimally fill up your lungs with oxygen, which is in demand as you challenge your muscles. Proper breathing also provides you with core stability, helps you to align your body, and, as an end result, prevents injury.

Should I stretch before or after strength training?

The answer is neither. Stretching before exercise is never recommended. Think of your muscles as cold rubber bands. What happens when you try to stretch the cold band? Odds are, it's going to possibly break or, at the very least, tear. The exact same thing occurs when you attempt to stretch a cold muscle. Now, the benefits of postexercise stretching are hotly debated. One group says you must stretch your muscles out after strength training. They believe that in order to build long, lean muscles, you must stretch them out before the tiny tears repair over the next twenty-four to forty-eight hours. The other side believes that a properly balanced strength-training program effectively stretches out the body. Let's again use the example of a bicep curl. When you curl up, you are simultaneously lengthening and stretching the triceps muscles. Right now, curl your arm up. Do you see how the triceps lengthened? When you perform strength training in a safe, controlled manner while working a full range of motion, you are effectively stretching the muscle opposite the one you are training. This is called reciprocal inhibition, and it is my recommendation. Do you remember back in Chapter 2 when I said that performing strength training gave you heart-health benefits and an increased metabolism? I referred to it as a "two birds with one stone" solution. When you add flexibility as one more benefit, it truly becomes a "three birds with one stone" phenomenon.

What about Pilates and yoga?

I have a love-hate relationship with both Pilates and yoga. Let's start with Pilates. I don't like the mat classes. It's just another class asking you to perform way too many repetitions without failure (the next chapter will explain this concept to you). Pilates performed on the Reformer and the Cadillac equipment can be an effective strength-training tool and can enhance posture and core strength, but the instructor must apply significant progression for it to be effective. The majority of instructors I have observed don't make the exercises hard enough to shock your muscles into growth.

Yoga has become extremely popular. For a true beginner, there is some benefit to your muscles when holding the poses. Similar to Pilates, there are also benefits to your posture. The problem comes when applying progression, since the only option is to hold the pose longer. You can't increase the weight or tension, because all the moves are done against your own body weight. Therefore, unless you are willing to increase the duration (find a longer class or double up) or the frequency (go more often each week), yoga alone won't get the job done. Both Pilates and yoga are good complements to a strength-training program, but on their own, they are not solutions for losing weight.

On a final note, celebrities (many of whom are paid) have been huge advocates of Pilates and yoga and have endlessly preached their benefits in print and in infomercials. The vast majority of these young women were very thin in the first place. How many women do you know who have truly lost weight simply with Pilates or yoga? I'm in the industry, and I don't know of any.

Glamour magazine reported the results of a Chicago versus New York versus Los Angeles challenge in its February 2005 issue. Every woman was placed on the same eating plan, but there were three different exercise plans. In L.A. it was Yoga Booty Balance class, which "combines fun, heart-pumping moves with a dash of yoga"; Pilates was the exercise in New York, led by a guru who has worked with the likes of Madonna and Uma Thurman; and in Chicago it was yours truly and strength training. Who won? Come on, would I mention this article if I didn't win? My group took it in a virtual landslide, with a total of fifty pounds and a whopping eighty-four inches lost. What was the secret? They performed heavy-duty strength training. And to this day, they have kept almost all of it off. One of the women just had her second baby and weighs *less* than she did before the first baby, and her pre-pregnancy jeans—before the first baby—are falling off.

CHAPTER 8

The Cardio-Free
Exercise Program

It's time to introduce you to the Cardio-Free Four-Phase Exercise Program. I have included two exercise plans, one with SPRI exercise tubing and one with free weights. Both are equally effective in maintaining and building long, lean, calorie-burning muscles. While both plans are easily executed in your home, office, or exercise facility, the plan using the SPRI exercise tubing is perfect while traveling.

I begin both routines with ten main exercises. Every two weeks, as you progress from Phase I to II to III and, ultimately, to IV, you will add two exercises to the original set of ten. This ensures that you continue to progress your plan, which is the true secret to effective exercise. Progression is the secret to success!

I have placed more emphasis on exercises that work the back of the body, because in life, we generally engage in activities that use the fronts of our bodies—only those who ride horses and row boats fully utilize their backs. To promote good posture and improve what we in the fitness industry call your "structural integrity," it is best to devote more time to your back, rear deltoid (back of the shoulder), lower back, gluteal, and hamstring muscles. If the muscles of your body are balanced and aligned properly, you will look and feel better, and you will be less prone to injury.

NOTE: In the past, men placed a great deal of emphasis on working their chest and bicep muscles under the assumption that this would make them look good. Just the opposite occurred: poor posture and muscular imbalance. Most men are surprised when I tell them that the key to a great chest is to work the back twice as often as the chest. Right now, pull your shoulders back. Didn't your chest just pop out? That is what will happen when you follow this exercise plan. The same applies to a man's desire to get bigger arms. The triceps muscles in the back of the arm actually account for two-thirds of the size of the arm. While men have thought working the bicep was going to give them good arms, it's actually triceps development that will create the most appealing visual.

The majority of the exercises in your Cardio-Free Exercise Program are known in the fitness industry as compound exercises. These use many muscle groups at the same time. They optimize the calories you burn during the time spent on the actual exercise, and they maximize the amount of lean muscle tissue you create. They also help with your heart-health benefits, because the more muscles we use, the more oxygen-rich blood is required.

To engage or recruit more muscle groups, all standing exercises in both Program 1 and Program 2 will be performed in what is referred to as a "staggered stance." By placing the right foot forward and the left foot back (the heel of the right foot is approximately one to one and a half feet in front of the toes of the left), you immediately engage more of the gluteal muscles, which are the largest muscles of the body and therefore will recruit more muscle fiber and oxygen during the workout. You also place more of a challenge on your core in this position. I will ask you to perform the first five reps with the right foot forward, then shift to the left foot forward for the last five reps.

In Phase I, the optimal speed of each repetition should be two counts on the concentric or lifting stage and four counts on the lengthening (eccentric) stage back to starting position. For a bicep curl, that would mean two counts as you curl up and four counts as you bring the weight back to your thighs. Given that you will perform ten reps, each set should take you approximately sixty seconds, or one minute. If you are finishing your set faster than that, then you know you need to slow down.

The moment you are finished with your set, immediately go on to the next exercise. If you quickly get a drink of water, record your weights/ tension and reps and prepare for the next exercise, you should never rest more than thirty seconds between each exercise.

Turn the page for a chart detailing the benefits of the Cardio-Free Exercise Program.

KEYS TO THE CARDIO-FREE EXERCISE PLAN	RESULT
1. Short, Intense Workouts	Saves Time
2. Interval Training	Promotes Heart Health
3. Always Going to Failure	Builds Muscle
4. Progressing Your Plan	Ensures Continued Success
5. Compound Movements	Burns Calories
6. Emphasis on Back	Improves Posture and Alignment
7. Slow Movement	Recruits More Muscle Fiber

Program 1—SPRI Exercise Tubing

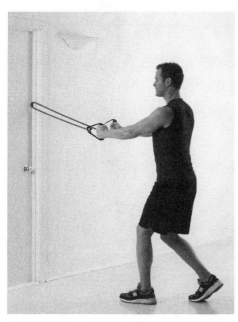

• Phase I (Weeks 1 and 2)

All standing exercises are performed in the stagger stance to engage the lower body. You will perform one set of each exercise to failure until instructed otherwise. For number of reps, number of sets, and amount of time per exercise, please see chapter 9.

The Ten Main Exercises

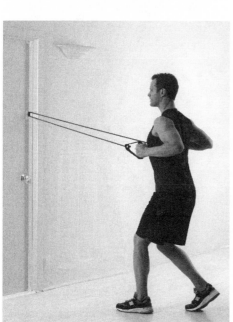

1. Back Row on Both Legs with the Xertube

a. Insert the Xertube into the door attachment, then attach it to the door, level with your chest.

b. Stand approximately four feet from the door with your feet in the stagger stance, your toes forward and abdominals tucked.

c. Grasp the Xertube with your palms facing each other and pull your shoulders back.

d. Slowly exhale as you pull the Xertube toward you and hold for two counts.

e. Concentrate on pulling your shoulder blades together.

f. Slowly inhale as you release.

NOTE: Make sure to stand upright at all times, and try not to lean back.

2. Hip Extension with the Lex Loop

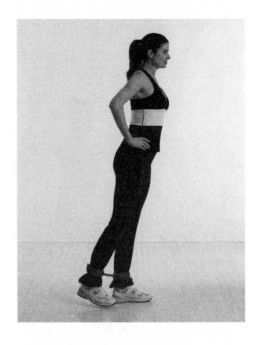

a. Place the Lex Loop around both ankles.

b. Place your arms on your hips or use a chair or wall for balance.

c. Shift your weight onto your left leg, and lift your right leg slightly off the floor.

d. Slowly exhale as you press your right leg back and hold for two counts.

e. Inhale as you return and keep your right leg off of the floor until all repetitions are completed.

f. Repeat using the left leg.

NOTE: Concentrate on your glutes (rear end) through-out the exercise; you will feel this exercise on both sides.

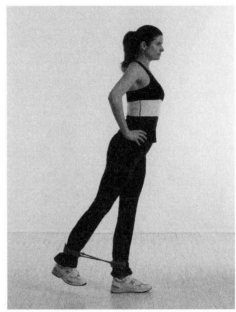

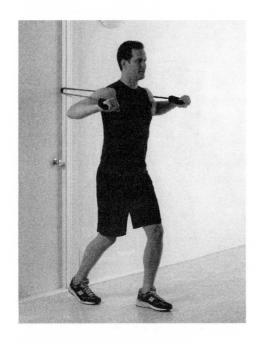

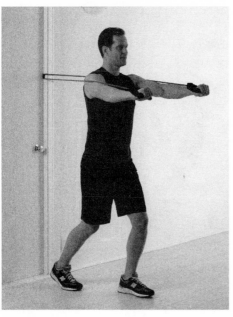

3. Chest Press on Both Legs with the Xertube

a. Attach the Xertube to the door.

b. Stand approximately four feet away with your back to the door in the stagger stance, with your toes facing forward and abdominals tucked.

c. Grasp the Xertube with your palms facing down.

d. Slowly exhale as you press the Xertube out while squeezing your chest.

e. Hold for two counts, then inhale as you release until your elbows are on the same plane as your shoulders.

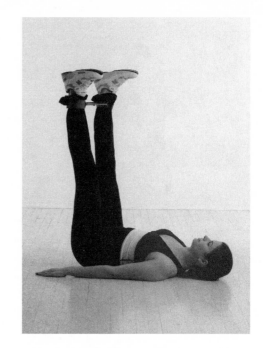

4. Lying-Down Hip Abduction with the Lex Loop

a. Lie on the ground with your legs up and the Lex Loop around both ankles.

b. Keep your head, neck, shoulders, and lower back firmly on the ground. (NOTE: Place a rolled towel under your neck if it bothers you in any way.)

c. With straight legs and flexed feet, slowly exhale as you press your feet out to your sides.

d. Hold for two counts, then slowly inhale as you return.

NOTE: The more tension you create, the more you will feel the effects of this exercise in your glutes and hips.

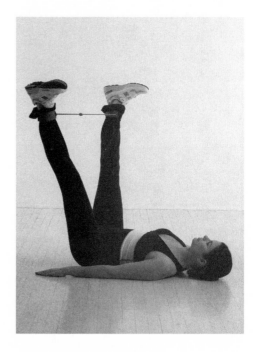

THE CARDIO-FREE DIET

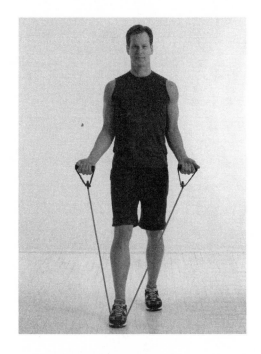

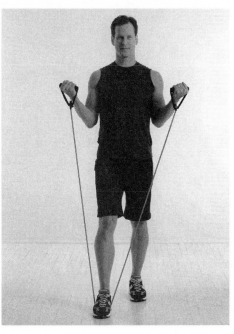

5. Bicep Curl with the Xertube

a. Stand in the stagger stance with your right foot forward and left foot back.

b. Place the Xertube under your right leg. Make sure to stand straight up, keeping your shoulders back and abdominals tucked.

c. Slowly exhale as you curl the Xertube toward you with your palms facing up.

d. Hold for two counts, then slowly inhale as you release back to the starting position, where the elbow is still slightly bent. The curl is finished when your elbow starts to move up from your side.

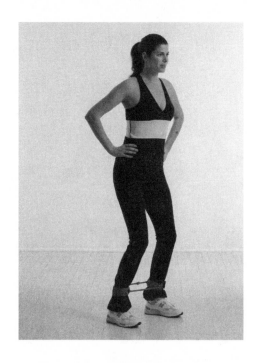

6. Drop-Step Abduction with the Lex Loop: "The Speed Skater"

a. Place the Lex Loop around both ankles.

b. Place your hands on your hips and assume the quarter-squat position.

c. Start with your feet together, then press your right leg out and back at a 45-degree angle and place your foot down and hold for two counts.

d. Slowly bring your right foot back to the starting position, then switch to your left leg. This movement should mimic the motion of a speed skater.

NOTE: At all times, stay in the quarter-squat position.

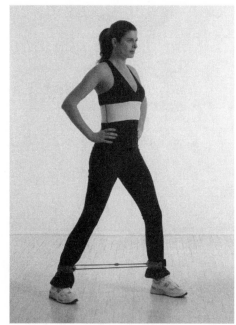

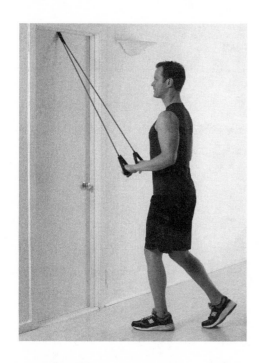

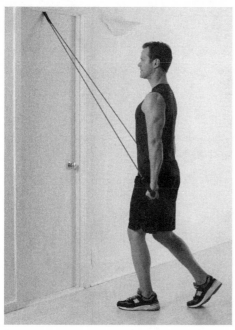

7. Tricep Pushdown with the Xertube

a. Insert the Xertube into the door attachment and secure it at the top of the door.

b. Stand in the stagger stance, with your toes forward and abdominals tucked.

c. Grasp the Xertube with your palms facing down and your elbows secured at your sides.

d. Slowly exhale as you press your arms down and hold for two counts, then inhale as you release.

NOTE: Be sure to concentrate on your triceps and squeeze them as you press the Xertube down.

8. Abdominal Crunch with the Xertube

a. Leave the Xertube attached at the top of the door as you did for the Tricep Pushdown.

b. Kneel down three feet away from the door with one Xertube handle in each hand.

c. Secure your arms at your sides, then slowly exhale as you curl your torso down and squeeze your abdominals.

d. Hold for two counts, then slowly inhale as you return to the starting position.

NOTE: Your hands and arms should never move from the starting position. Only your torso curls forward to engage the abdominals.

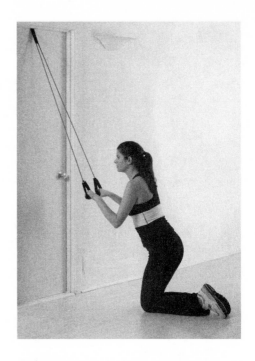

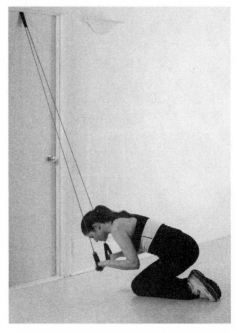

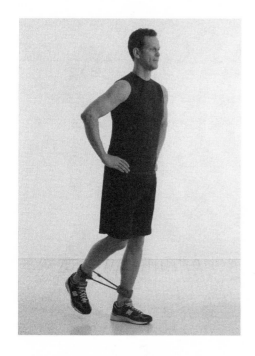

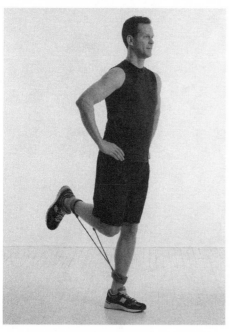

9. Standing Hamstring Curl with the Lex Loop

a. Stand with the Lex Loop around both ankles.

b. Shift your weight onto your left leg and slowly lift your right leg behind you with your toes flexed.

c. Exhale as you slowly curl your right foot up toward your right glute.

d. Hold for two counts, then inhale as you lower your leg to starting position.

NOTE: Maintain perfect posture and keep your abdominals tucked at all times. You should also feel this in the support leg.

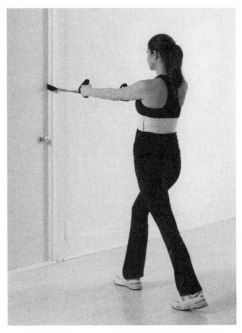

10. Rear Deltoid Fly on Both Legs with the Xertube

a. Insert the Xertube into the door attachment, then attach it to the door, level with your chest.

b. Stand in the stagger stance, with your toes forward and abdominals tucked.

c. Grasp the Xertube with your palms facing each other and pull your shoulders back.

d. Slowly exhale as you pull the Xertube out to both sides and then back with slightly bent arms. This is a fly movement, not a row, as in the first exercise.

e. Hold for two counts, then slowly inhale as you return to the starting position.

NOTE: Make sure to stand upright at all times and to not lean back.

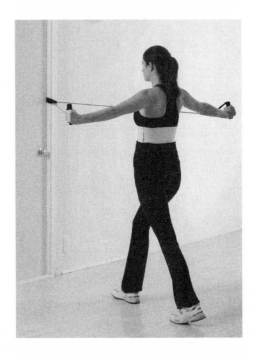

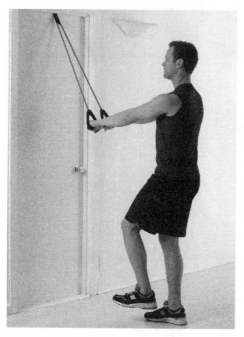

• Phase II (Weeks 3 and 4)

Add these exercises for a total of twelve exercises. You will perform a second set of half of the exercises. Therefore, your first session, you will perform two sets of exercises 1–6 and one set of exercises 7–12. The next time you work out, perform one set of exercises 1–6 and two sets of exercises 7–12. Keep alternating throughout the phase.

11. Straight-Arms Pushdown on One Leg with the Xertube

NOTE: This is the first exercise that requires you to stand on one leg instead of two.

a. Attach the Xertube to the top of the door.

b. Stand about three feet from the door on your right foot with your left foot lifted up.

c. Grasp the Xertube with an overhand grip, your arms fully extended.

d. Slowly inhale, then exhale as you press your arms straight down to your sides.

e. Hold for two counts, then inhale as you return to starting position.

NOTE: This is a straight-arm movement, which is different from the Tricep Pushdown, where the arms were bent at the elbows.

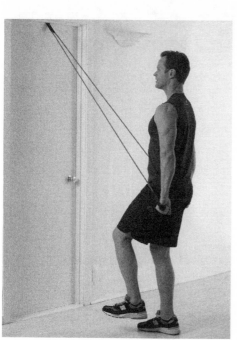

THE CARDIO-FREE EXERCISE PROGRAM

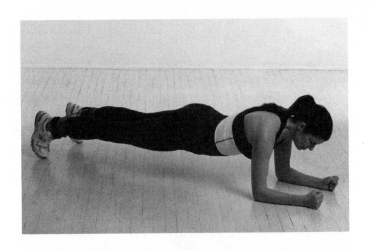

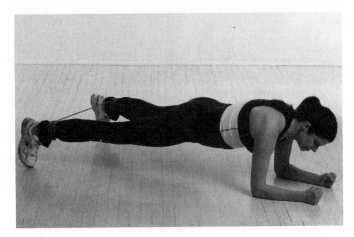

12. Plank with the Lex Loop at the Ankles

a. Place the Lex Loop around both ankles and assume the plank position on your elbows.

b. Make sure to keep your abdominals tucked at all times.

c. Once you have assumed the plank and held it for fifteen seconds, press your legs out as far as they can go and hold for another fifteen seconds.

d. Return legs to original position, and repeat the exercise two additional times.

NOTE: The key is to keep your back as flat as possible, as that will optimally challenge your abs while simultaneously working your upper and lower body.

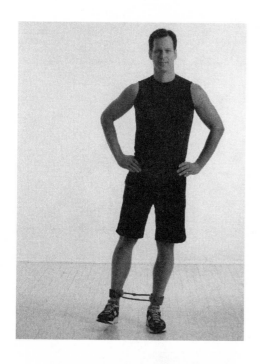

• Phase III (Weeks 5 and 6)

Add these exercises for a total of fourteen. Similar to Phase II, you will perform a second set of half of the exercises. Therefore, your first session you will perform two sets of exercises 1–7 and one set of exercises 8–14. The next time you work out, you will perform one set of exercises 1–7 and two sets of exercises 8–14. Continue alternating throughout the phase.

13. Standing Hip Abduction with the Lex Loop

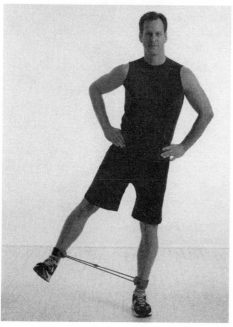

a. Place the Lex Loop around both ankles.

b. Place your hands on your hips, or use a chair or wall for balance.

c. Shift your weight onto your left leg; lift your right leg slightly off the floor and flex your toes up.

d. Slowly exhale as you press your right leg out to the side and hold for two counts.

e. Inhale as you return. (NOTE: Keep your right leg off the floor until all repetitions are completed.)

f. Repeat using your left leg.

NOTE: Concentrate on both your glutes and hips throughout the exercise, as you will be working them both.

14. Lateral Raise with the Xertube in the Lunge Position

a. Assume a lunge position with your left foot forward and right foot back.

b. Both feet should face forward and your abdominals should be tucked.

c. Place the Xertube under your left foot.

d. Bend all the way down into the low position of the lunge, then begin to slowly perform a lateral raise.

e. Exhale as you lift the Xertube to shoulder height, hold for two counts, then inhale as you return to the starting position.

f. If you have to, switch legs after five reps—if not, then make a note of which leg you had in front, and use your other leg the next time you perform the exercise.

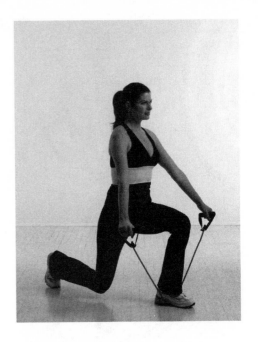

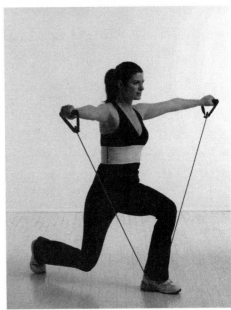

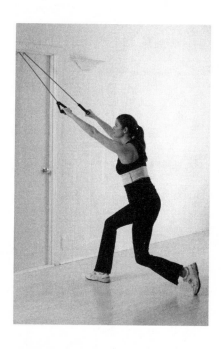

• Phase IV (Weeks 7 and 8)

Add these two exercises for a total of sixteen. In Phase IV, you will perform two sets of each exercise.

15. Lat Pulldown with the Xertube

a. Attach the Xertube to the top of the door.

b. Assume a near-lunge position, keeping your legs slightly closer together than you would in the lunge position.

c. Grasp the Xertube with an overhead grip.

d. Slowly exhale as you pull the handles down to your sides.

e. Hold for two counts, then inhale as you slowly release the handles back up to starting position.

NOTE: Concentrate on your lats (back muscles), biceps, and lower back, and make sure your lower body stays in the same position throughout the exercise.

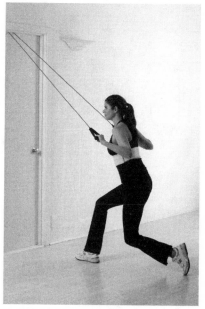

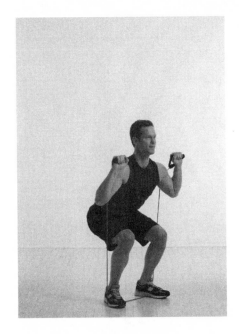

16. Shoulder Press in the Squat Position with the Xertube

a. Stand with your feet shoulder-width apart and your toes forward.

b. Place the Xertube under both feet, with the handles facing forward at your shoulders.

c. Inhale as you slowly lower yourself into a squat position, with your hamstrings almost parallel with the floor.

d. Exhale as you lift up from the squat, pressing your arms up into a shoulder press, and hold for two counts.

NOTE: Make sure that your hands never fall below shoulder height.

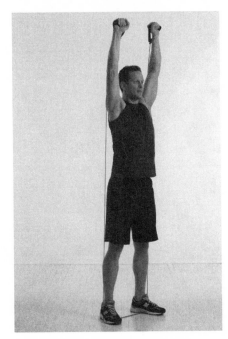

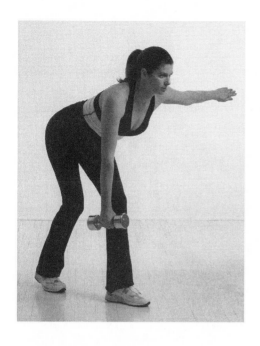

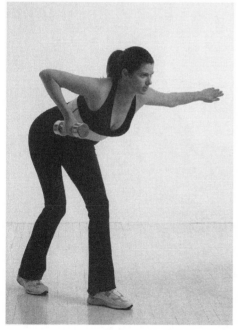

Program 2—Free Weights

• Phase I (Weeks 1 and 2)

All standing exercises are performed in the stagger stance to engage the lower body. You will perform one set of each exercise to failure until instructed otherwise.

The Ten Main Exercises

1. One-Arm Row

a. Place your feet in the stagger stance.

b. With a dumbbell in your right hand, hold your left arm straight out at your side.

c. Keep your head and chin aligned as pictured.

d. As you exhale, slowly pull the dumbbell up until it almost touches your chest and hold for two counts.

e. Inhale as you release, but keep your elbow slightly bent at the bottom.

NOTE: Tuck in your abdominals at all times to support your lower back, and make sure that you are only lifting your arm and not your working shoulder. You should progress quickly in weight on this exercise. I alluded to this earlier, on page 44.

2. Stationary Lunges

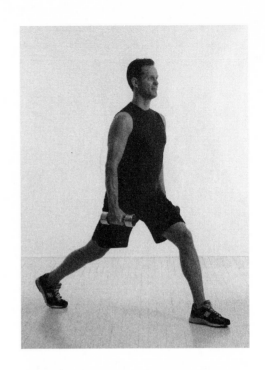

a. Stand with your feet approximately three feet apart, with your left foot forward and your right foot back.

b. Both feet should face forward, and your back heel should be up at all times.

c. Hold the dumbbells at your sides with your palms facing in. (NOTE: Beginners may elect to start without using dumbbells.)

d. Slowly inhale as you lower your body into the lunge position, bending both knees, and hold for two counts.

e. Exhale as you lift back up, squeezing your left glute.

f. Make sure your forward knee never passes your forward toes.

g. Your back knee should end up approximately three inches off the floor.

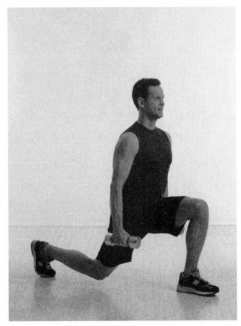

NOTE: You should continue to increase the amount of weight as long as you can complete the ten repetitions.

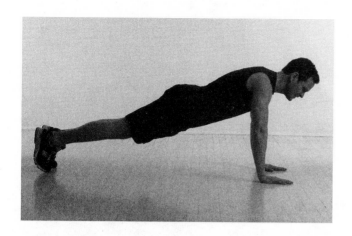

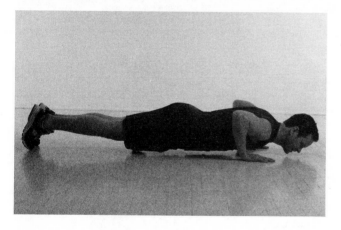

3. Push-up

a. Place your hands shoulder-width apart with your fingertips spread.

b. For beginners, start on your knees with your toes down (not up and crossed)—if you feel more advanced, go ahead and start at your toes (you can always drop down to finish the set).

c. Inhale as you lower down to two inches off the ground; hold for two counts, then slowly exhale as you press up.

NOTE: Make sure to keep your abdominals tucked at all times to support your lower back.

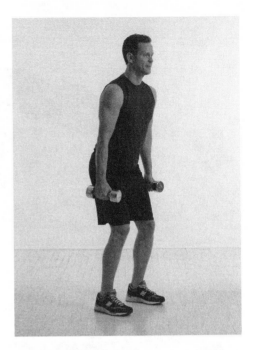

4. Squat

a. Stand with your feet shoulder-width apart and your toes forward, with soft knees.

b. Place a dumbbell in each hand, with your palms facing your hips.

c. Pull your shoulders back and down, and maintain this straight back throughout the movement.

d. Slowly sit back into your heels and bend slightly forward to balance your body.

e. Make sure your knees never extend past your toes.

f. Ideally, the end of the movement occurs when your hamstrings are parallel with the floor.

g. Inhale on the way down, hold for two counts, then exhale on the way back up to starting position.

NOTE: Really concentrate on your glutes and squeeze them as you lift—remember, link the mind to the muscle.

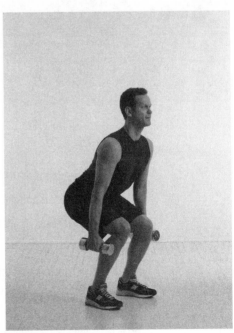

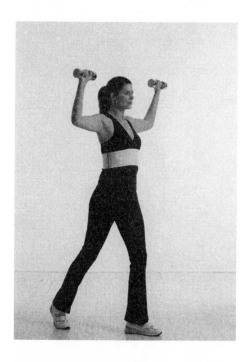

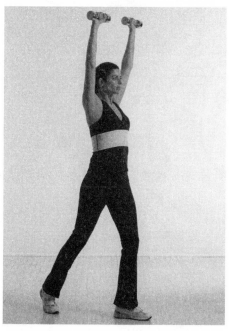

5. Shoulder Press

a. Place your feet in the stagger stance.

b. Place a dumbbell in each hand and begin with your elbows on the same plane as your shoulders.

c. Palms should face forward at all times.

d. Slowly exhale as you press the weights straight up over your head.

e. Hold for two counts, then slowly inhale as you return to the starting position.

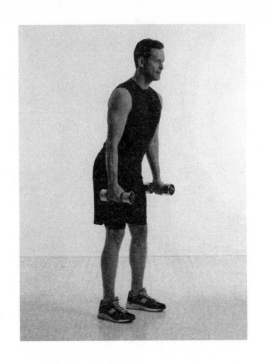

6. Dead Lift

a. Stand with your feet shoulder-width apart and your toes forward, with soft knees.

b. Place a dumbbell in each hand, with your palms facing your hips.

c. Pull your shoulders back and down, and maintain this straight back throughout the movement.

d. Slowly bend from the hips—*not* your lower back—until you feel a full stretch in your hamstrings.

e. Inhale on the way down, hold for two counts, then exhale on the way up.

NOTE: Keep your weight always in your heels, and make sure that the dumbbells track straight down your legs. Stop if you feel any pain in your lower back.

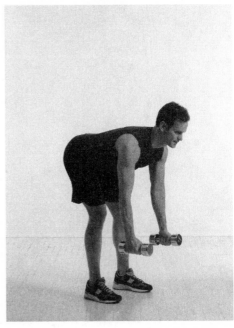

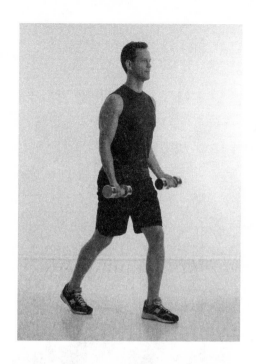

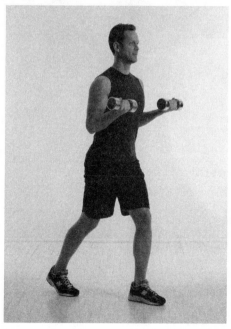

7. Bicep Curl

a. Place your feet in the stagger stance.

b. Place a dumbbell in each hand at your thighs, palms facing forward, elbows at your sides.

c. Slowly exhale as you curl each weight up until your elbows start to move away from your body, and hold for two counts.

d. Inhale as you return the weights to the starting position, but maintain a slight bend to keep the tension.

NOTE: You will quickly progress to using heavier weights, which is good!

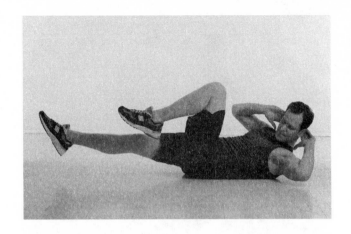

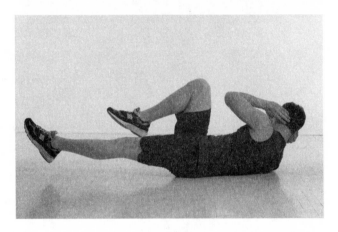

8. Abdominal Bicycle

a. Lie on the ground with your legs straight out in front of you and your hands at the sides of your head.

b. Slowly pull your left knee toward you and lift your right leg just two inches off the floor.

c. Lift your right shoulder—not elbow—toward your left leg.

d. Hold for two counts, then switch to the other side.

e. Count one rep as working both the right and left side ten times, for a total of twenty movements.

NOTE: If you feel this at all in your back, lift the extended leg higher.

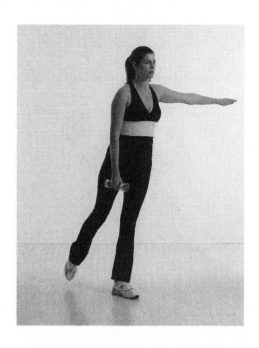

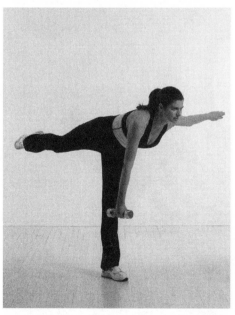

9. One-Leg Reach

a. Balance on your left leg and hold a dumbbell in your right hand, palm facing inward.

b. Slowly, with tucked abdominals and a flat back, begin to reach with your right arm toward the left foot.

c. The key is to keep your body perfectly straight.

d. Inhale on the way down, hold for two counts, and exhale as you return to the starting position.

NOTE: If you need to start without a dumbbell or need to hold on to a chair or wall for support, that is just fine.

10. Bent-Over Rear Deltoid Fly

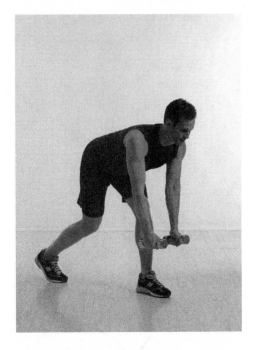

a. Place your feet in the stagger stance.

b. Hold a light dumbbell in each hand, as this is a difficult exercise.

c. Slowly exhale as you lift the weights out to your side and hold for two counts.

d. Keep your arms almost fully extended with just a slight bend in your elbows.

e. Inhale as you return to starting position.

f. Maintain a flat back as much as possible by tucking your abdominals.

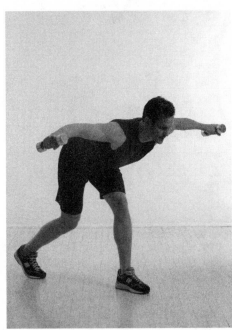

THE CARDIO-FREE DIET

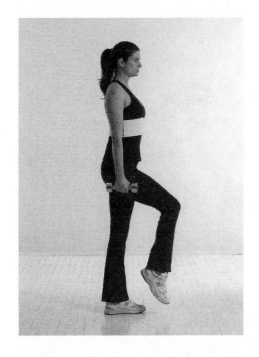

• Phase II (Weeks 3 and 4)

Add these exercises for a total of twelve exercises. You will perform a second set of half of the exercises. Therefore, your first session, you will perform two sets of exercises 1–6 and one set of exercises 7–12. The next time you exercise, perform one set of exercises 1–6 and two sets of exercises 7–12. Continue alternating throughout the phase.

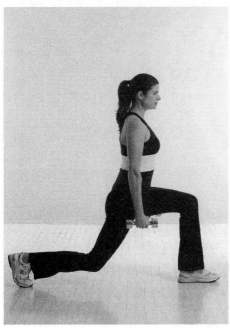

11. Back-Stepping Lunges

a. Start with your feet shoulder-width apart with your toes forward and abdominals tucked.

b. Slowly balance on your left leg as you reach back with the right.

c. Plant your right foot down as you go directly into a lunge.

d. Pause for two counts, then bring the right leg back to the starting position.

e. Inhale as you reach back, exhale as you return.

f. Keep your abdominals tucked at all times.

g. Perform ten reps with your right leg stepping back, then perform ten using your left, for twenty reps total.

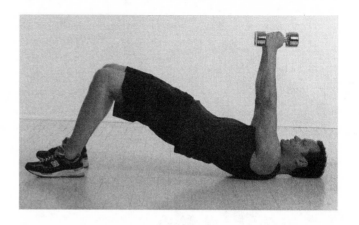

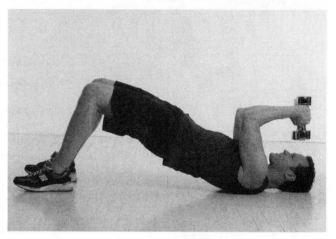

12. Lying-Down Tricep Extension While Bridging

a. Lie on your back with your legs bent and your feet firmly planted on the floor, about shoulder-width apart.

b. Place one dumbbell in each hand and extend your arms over your chest.

c. Your palms should face each other at all times and your wrists should stay in alignment.

d. Before you begin to lower the weights, lift your hips up into a bridge position to engage your glutes, hamstrings, lower back, and abdominals.

e. Slowly inhale as you lower the dumbbells alongside your ears, hold for two counts, then exhale as you press your arms back up to the starting position.

NOTE: Keep your abdominals tucked at all times to support your lower back.

THE CARDIO-FREE DIET

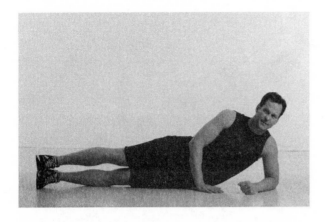

• **Phase III (Weeks 5 and 6)**
Add these exercises for a total of fourteen. Similar to Phase II, you will perform a second set of half of the exercises. Therefore, your first session, you will perform two sets of exercises 1–7 and one set of exercises 8–14. The next time you exercise, you will perform one set of exercises 1–7 and two sets of exercises 8–14. Continue alternating throughout the phase.

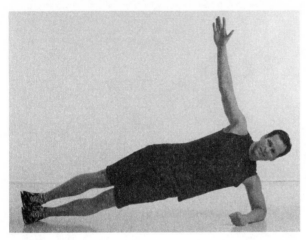

13. Side Plank

a. Lie on your side with your right leg directly on top of your left.

b. Both feet should be flexed at all times.

c. Lift yourself up onto your left elbow and place your right hand directly in front of you for balance.

d. Slowly lift up your body, ideally creating a straight diagonal line, and reach your palm up with your arm forward.

e. Hold for fifteen seconds, then come down and rest for another fifteen. Repeat on the same side, then switch.

f. Your goal should always be time, so make sure to have a clock or watch handy.

NOTE: You should ultimately progress to holding for one minute on each side.

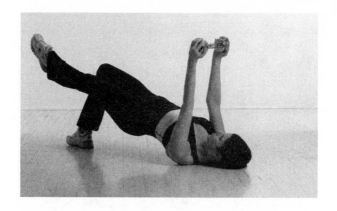

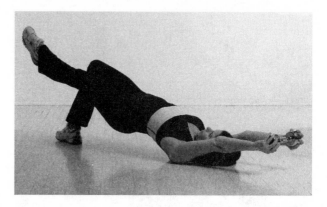

14. Bridge Pullover

a. Lie on your back with your right leg planted and left leg extended, with a pointed toe.

b. Place one dumbbell in each hand and extend your arms over your head.

c. Palms should face each other at all times and your wrists should stay aligned.

d. Before you begin to lower the weights, lift your hips up into the bridge position to engage your glutes, hamstrings, lower back, and abdominals.

e. Slowly inhale as you lower the dumbbells with your arms straight along each side of your head, then exhale as you press your arms back up to the starting position.

f. Keep your abdominals tucked at all times to support your lower back.

NOTE: This is a straight-arm movement and is different than the Tricep Extension, where the arms were bent at the elbows.

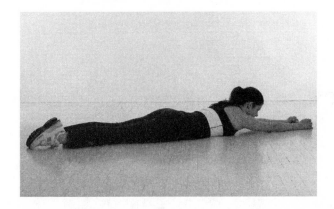

• Phase IV (Weeks 7 and 8)
Add these two exercises for a total of sixteen. In Phase IV, you will perform two sets of each exercise.

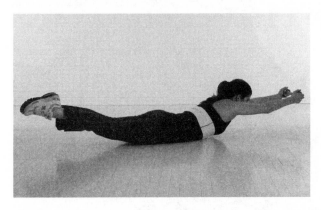

15. Superman

a. Lie prone with your arms and legs completely extended.

b. Place one light dumbbell in both hands, holding it with your palms facing each other.

c. Slowly inhale, then exhale as you simultaneously lift both your arms and legs.

d. Hold for two counts, then return to the starting position.

e. With each rep, attempt to lift up higher.

NOTE: Keep your chin in a neutral position as shown and rest if you feel any tension.

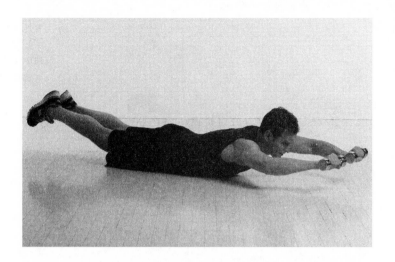

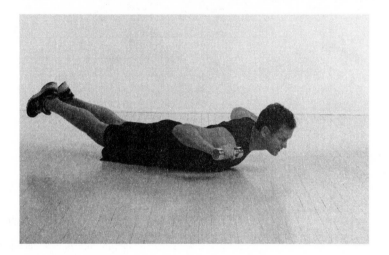

16. Prone Pulldown

a. Assume the same position as you did for the Superman exercise.

b. Place one light dumbbell in each hand with your palm facing down.

c. Inhale as you lift up into the starting position pictured.

d. Slowly exhale as you pull the weights down to your sides.

e. Hold for two counts, then return to the starting position.

NOTE: This is a difficult exercise, so you may need to start without weights.

CHAPTER 9

How to Progress Your Cardio-Free Exercise Program

In Chapter 2, I mentioned that you have to keep increasing either the frequency, intensity, or duration of your cardiovascular exercise in order to keep burning the same number of calories. I also explained that as you increase the intensity, frequency, or duration of cardiovascular activity, you also increase your risk of injury by overusing your muscles, tendons, ligaments, and joints. In strength training, you must also keep challenging your muscles to grow, which we call progression.

The difference between a strength-training program and a cardiovascular exercise program is that progressing your strength training is much safer and ultimately more effective. Your body craves strength training, as possessing more muscle makes everything easier. Having more muscle also preserves your joints, tendons, and ligaments and ultimately serves to make you feel and look younger. With progressive strength training, you are helping your body to change and improve, whereas increasing cardio ultimately breaks your body down.

Many people neglect to apply progression to their strength-training routine. That is why they hit a plateau and, in most instances, discontinue the program for lack of results. Women, especially, are reluctant to increase the tension/weight for fear of getting too big. But the most significant benefits of strength training come to those who do apply progression effectively.

I said in Chapter 4 that for seniors,

If You Don't Lift, You Don't Last

For all of us, seniors included,

If You Don't Progress, You May Regress

Skipping the progression will most likely result in an end to your strength training and a return to your body's former composition, both internally and externally. Don't let that happen.

You can progress your strength and resistance training program in a number of ways:

- Increase the weight.

- Increase the reps.

- Increase the sets.

- Slow down the speed of each rep and increase the time under tension.

- Stand farther away from the door attachment.

- Lower your staggered stance.

- Change your hand position.

- Add instability.

- Switch programs.

Let's take a look at these, one at a time.

INCREASE THE WEIGHT

This is probably the simplest and most effective way (especially in the beginning) to progress your strength and resistance program. After you can accomplish ten reps of a particular exercise without achieving failure, you must increase the weight or tension. You should always increase with the smallest increment possible, both to help avoid injury and to progress consistently. With free weights, that would mean going from the five-pound dumbbells (which should be used only for a few exercises, such as the rear deltoid fly, as they are too light for everything else) to the eights, then tens, twelves, fifteens, and so on. With the SPRI exercise tubing, that would mean going from yellow (which is actually too light for most people) to green, red, blue, and ultimately purple.

When you raise the tension, don't feel that you should be able to perform all ten reps right away. Instead, do as many with proper form as you can. Then you may choose to execute what is called a "drop set" or "extended set," where you perform the first four, six, or eight reps with the twelve-pound dumbbells, then drop back to the tens to finish the last reps. This is a perfectly acceptable and smart way to progress. Don't expect to jump to an increased weight/tension and be able to finish a set of ten reps. Remember that most people fall off a workout program after injuring themselves, which happens when they go at it too intensely or progress too quickly.

INCREASE THE REPS

We have all heard people say, "You should do heavy weights and low reps to build muscle, and light weights and high reps to tone." This is completely wrong. High repetitions of low weights do nothing to build your muscles, because your muscles never reach failure. Most research indicates that increasing the reps means overutilizing your joints. Similar to excessive cardio, excessive repetitions with strength training may break you down rather than build you up. The best way to stimulate muscle growth while protecting and strengthening your joints is to go heavier with fewer reps.

INCREASE THE SETS

The number of sets is really a function of the time you have to dedicate to exercise. One set to failure is excellent for beginners, and even some more advanced individuals will see great results with only one set.

NOTE: If you plan to strength train on back-to-back days, doing all upper body one day and lower the next, double your sets, since you are performing only half as many exercises.

For Phases II and III, I ask you to go to two sets for half of the exercises. For Phase IV, I ask you to go to two sets for each exercise. This progression will allow you to achieve optimal results in the eight-week time period.

SLOW DOWN THE SPEED OF EACH REP

I like the concept of slowing down, as most people lift weights with reckless abandon, and that's exactly what I don't want you to do. Start your strength-training program with two counts on the contraction (one, one thousand, two, one thousand) and four counts on the return. Because your muscles are stronger on the eccentric (or lowering phase) of any strength-training movement, I want you to always spend at least double the time on the eccentric as the concentric part of the movement. To progress, go to a three-count on the way up and a six-count on the way down, or a four-count on the way up and an eight-count on the way down, until you get to a five-count on the way up and a ten count on the way down. That is as slow as you should go. This is a very safe way for people of all ages to progress, but is especially applicable to the senior population. You want to preserve your joints at any cost, and the slower you go, the less stress will be placed on your joints, and the more will be placed on your muscles and bones. And make sure you don't just start counting faster!

STAND FARTHER AWAY FROM THE DOOR ATTACHMENT

For any of the exercises done with the SPRI Xertube and the door attachment, standing farther away from the door is going to increase the intensity of the exercise. I urge you to generally adopt this strategy before going up to the next level of tension. When you are documenting your progress each session, simply make a notation as to how far away from the door your forward foot is standing. By moving that back, you are making the exercise harder. When you do feel you have gotten as far back as is comfortable, then it is time to go up to the next level of tension.

LOWER YOUR STAGGERED STANCE

One way to progress your plan is to lower your staggered stance for all of the standing exercises. Think of it as a partial lunge. By lowering the stance, you immediately place more tension on the lower body and core as you are performing the upper-body exercises. Trust me, you will feel it in your lower-body muscles and core and may find that you have to come back to a more upright position after the first few reps. That is fine. It is exactly like the dropped or extended set I described earlier. Don't expect to be able to lower the staggered stance and perform all ten repetitions the first time out.

CHANGE YOUR HAND POSITION

For all of the standing exercises for the lower body with the Lex Loop, such as the hip extension, hip abduction, and speed skater, changing your hand position will increase the intensity of the exercise. You can either raise your hands directly over your head or adopt what we call the "prison stance," by placing your hands to the side of your head with your elbows out. By placing your hands over your head, you immediately put more muscles into play and generally increase your heart rate. I am particularly partial to the prison stance, as it stretches out the chest and shoulder, an area that gets overused at the computer, while driving, and when carrying groceries, a purse, a briefcase, or luggage. That's why we are devoting twice as much time to the back of the body as the front.

ADD INSTABILITY

When you perform any of the standing strength-training exercises in the two programs, I have instructed you to stand on both feet in a staggered stance position. A great way to progress a standing exercise, such as the back row, is to stand on only one leg and lift the other off the floor.

If you elect to add instability, you should perform the first five reps on the right leg and then switch to the left for the remaining reps. You may find that you have to come down in tension/weight when you perform the exercises on one leg, since this will increase the overall difficulty of the exercise. When you perform any of the standing exercises on one leg, you immediately engage your core *and* you bring many more stabilizer muscles into play that support each main muscle group and help you to stay balanced. By recruiting all of these tiny stabilizer muscles that surround your major muscle groups, you enhance the lean, toned look that is so naturally appealing and sexy.

BOSU balls, which look like exercise balls cut in half, are an instability tool. By standing on either the round part on the top or by turning it over and working on the flat surface, you apply progression to your strength-training program. The same applies to the SPRI Xerdisc, which looks like a small plastic flying saucer and can be used for upper-body, lower-body, and core exercises.

If you work out at home, purchasing one of these instability tools will make sense for you at some point. The SPRI Xerdisc, in particular, is a favorite and is one-quarter the price of the BOSU. The SPRI Xerdisc can be used with almost every exercise in the two programs to apply progression. Just sitting on the Xerdisc at your desk or kitchen table (place it on top of the chair) forces you to use your core and promotes good posture.

SWITCH PROGRAMS

I purposely gave you two different programs so that you could alternate between them. After your first eight-week program, you may decide to go from the free-weight program to the one with the SPRI exercise tubing. That way, you shock your muscles with new stimuli. Most important, look at your schedule and plan accordingly. If this is going to be a heavy travel time, then by all means do the SPRI exercise program, since it is so easily transportable.

CHAPTER 10

The Cardio-Free Eating Rules

There has never been more confusion in the diet marketplace, and two strong camps have been battling it out for a number of years: the high-carbohydrate, low-fat group led by experts such as Dr. Dean Ornish and Dr. Nathan Pritikin; and the high-protein, low-carbohydrate group led by the late Dr. Robert Atkins and, more recently, Dr. Arthur Agatston of The South Beach Diet.

I want to help you make sense of all the confusion. Let's go over a few very important Cardio-Free eating rules and facts.

THERE ARE NO FORBIDDEN FOODS

I know from personal experience that the moment I am told not to eat a certain food, I start dreaming about it at night. Most research indicates that when you restrict a certain food group, all your body and mind want to do is eat it. It's basic human nature to want something you can't have. The moment you go on a "diet" in which you plan to eat one way for a particular period of time, hoping to get to a specific weight, and then plan to go back to "normal" eating once you've attained that weight, you have already doomed yourself to fail. To truly lose weight and keep it off, you must find a way to eat that you can stick with forever.

COUNT CALORIES

According to the Centers for Disease Control and Prevention, women are consuming 335 additional calories per day, which is approximately 20 percent more than they did back in 1971. If you crunch the numbers, 335 more calories a day will result in about thirty-five pounds of weight gain a year. Men are taking in only 168 more calories per day, which will result in a weight gain of (only!) seventeen and a half pounds each year.

The reason is what I call "portion distortion." We are consuming far too many calories on a daily basis, because the portion size of almost everything keeps growing. Have you read the bestseller *French Women Don't Get Fat*? The French eat far smaller portions of everything. When you take the portion size down, you immediately take the calorie count down. It's that simple. But in America, where bigger is always better, you actually have to leave some food on the plate (or take it home to eat tomorrow) to be able to walk, rather than roll, away.

When it comes to dieting, the calorie is more important than anything else. Researchers at Stanford and Yale universities analyzed 107 studies on low-carbohydrate diets, which have been around for the past thirty-five years. They found that the amount of carbohydrates consumed was not the determining factor in subjects who successfully lost weight. What mattered was the fact that most of the successful diets comprised around 1,100 calories.

EAT RIGHT BEFORE <u>AND</u> RIGHT AFTER EXERCISE

If you get up in the morning and exercise without eating, you are actually burning amino acids for fuel. And what tissue in the body is made up of amino acids? Muscle, which is why you must never, ever exercise without eating first. If you decide to exercise first thing in the morning, then you should eat half of your breakfast before your strength training and the other half after the workout. Regardless of the time of day, always eat before exercise in order to:

- ensure that glycogen (fuel) is available to perform the strength training optimally.

- make sure your blood sugar is up, so you have the mental and physical energy to strength train effectively.

- guarantee that your body will not burn amino acids (muscle) for fuel.

The perfect food choices (all about 100 calories) prior to exercise would include:

- a piece or serving (one cup cut up) of fruit

- a slice of whole wheat toast

- a cup of yogurt

- one packet of oatmeal

- half of your favorite two-hundred-calorie energy bar

- a half serving of a high-fiber cereal with low-fat milk

- half an apple with one teaspoon of peanut or apple butter

Your post-workout meal is very important to maximizing the benefits of the strength training you have just performed. There is something referred to as "the carbohydrate window." Basically, you want to replenish your muscles' glycogen storage tanks (think of them as small, individual gas tanks that power your muscles) as soon as you finish your strength training.

Post-workout, you always want to consume some protein with your carbohydrate. Proteins and amino acids are the building blocks of lean muscle tissue, and because the muscle repair process starts immediately, you want to make sure that you are not breaking down one muscle to repair another.

Post-workout options include:

- a slice of toast with cottage cheese, yogurt, or one piece of string cheese

- the other half of your favorite protein or energy bar

- one piece of fruit and one cup of yogurt

- oatmeal (one or two packets depending on the brand)

- a bowl of high-fiber, protein-enriched cereal and low-fat milk

- rolled-up turkey with a few whole wheat crackers

I want to be clear that the eating before and after exercise is essential to optimizing your results. When Hugh Jackman and I trained prior to his filming *X-Men: The Last Stand*, I made sure he ate on the way to the session and almost immediately after we were done working out. I know that this very specific eating plan was the reason he achieved such exceptional results with the strength training.

ALWAYS EAT BREAKFAST

The University of Massachusetts Medical School in Worcester reported that "people who regularly skipped breakfast were a whopping 450 percent more likely to be obese than regular breakfast eaters." The researchers added, "A lifestyle pattern that doesn't include breakfast is frequently associated with being overweight." Other researchers claim that those who frequently skip breakfast diminish their basal metabolism anywhere from 5 to 10 percent. Look at how much you can reduce your chances of being overweight just by doing what your mother always told you to do.

Research from the University of Texas at El Paso has shown that eating breakfast "proves more satiating than the same number of calories consumed later on and blunts overall calorie consumption." You will actually consume fewer calories over the entire day, because calories eaten earlier in the day make you feel fuller throughout the rest of the day. This study goes on to point out that as the day goes on, the time between meals diminishes. You wake up and have breakfast at seven a.m., then generally don't eat lunch until noon. That's five hours between breakfast and lunch. Around three thirty p.m., you are hungry for a snack. That's only three and a half hours. By six o'clock, you are ready for dinner (two and a half hours) and then at seven thirty, you are picking again (an hour and a half). And you know that most people don't stop snacking by seven thirty. Clearly your satiety mechanisms are diminishing as the day goes on.

So eat a good, solid breakfast with the right carbohydrates (fruits, vegetables, and whole grains) and protein. I will give you a number of tasty options in your Cardio-Free Eating Plan in the following chapter.

NEVER SKIP MEALS

Almost every client I have worked with over the past twenty years has come clean and told me that, in the past, they skipped meals as a strategy to lose weight. I always ask, "Did it work?" and they say, "Well, of course not, but I was desperate and skipping was all I could wrap a thought around."

Skipping leads to low blood sugar. Low blood sugar leads to low energy levels, possible dizziness, and then to a big binge. Have you ever awoken from a nap ravenous? It was because your blood sugar had dropped, and to bring it back into equilibrium, you ate—a lot, and fast! You are starving, so your body instructs you to get as much food in as possible. Plus, given the low blood sugar, nine times out of ten, you reach for something sweet, or something that will quickly turn to sugar in your body, like a simple carbohydrate. Using a "skip meals" strategy is a recipe for disaster. Like cardio, we've all tried it again and again in the past, and it just doesn't work.

While on the subject of skipping, let's address fasting. Fasting can lead to as much as *one pound of muscle loss each day*. As we've established, lean muscle is our most valuable asset in the fight for long-term weight loss, and losing a pound of muscle a day is the single biggest disaster fathomable. Don't sabotage yourself!

EAT THREE MEALS AND THREE SNACKS EACH DAY

Pacing your caloric intake throughout the day helps to keep you full and minimizes the chance of a binge. What is more efficient, throwing all the logs in the fire at once and hoping that they will burn all day, or slowly adding another log when one is just about burned out? Just as the second strategy will ensure a continual fire, pacing meals and snacks throughout the day will result in an optimized metabolism.

EAT PROTEIN AT EVERY MEAL

Don't think I am going Atkins on you—I'm not. High-protein, high-fat, low-carbohydrate eating plans are not healthy for you. Some of the crazier low-carbohydrate and high-protein diets ask for up to 60 percent of all calories to come from protein. That makes absolutely no sense. Your body *needs* carbohydrates, and the most nutritious foods—fruits, vegetables, and whole grains—are all carbohydrates. Your brain functions on carbohydrates, and they are essential to your body. But protein is the most difficult food to digest, and it will keep you feeling full longer. It will also help preserve your body's muscle. The Cardio-Free Eating Plan recommends 30 percent protein as the goal.

A study conducted at the University of Illinois at Urbana–Champaign placed two groups of women on a 1,700-calorie diet. Those who consumed 30 percent of their calories from protein lost more weight than those consuming only 15 percent. Donald K. Layman, the lead author, says that "eating more protein will increase the amount of the amino acid leucine in your diet, helping to maintain muscle mass during weight loss." A similar study from the Harvard School of Public Health placed three groups of people on very specific eating plans that had the exact same number of calories. The winning plan, with an average of twenty-three pounds lost, was the plan in which 30 percent of calories consumed came from protein. It resulted in six additional pounds of weight loss over the higher-carbohydrate, lower-protein plan.

Digestion actually burns calories and can account for between 5 and 10 percent of your basal metabolism. The calorie-burning process of digestion is called the thermogenic effect of food and occurs as protein is reduced to amino acids, carbohydrates to simple sugars, and fats to fatty acids. Protein has a higher thermogenic effect than carbs, and carbs have a higher effect than fat. Most research indicates that it takes as much as 30 percent of the caloric value of protein to break it down during digestion. That means that 100 protein calories will take about 30 calories to break down to amino acids and provide only 70 calories for use by the body. For the record, fat only requires 2 calories per 100 consumed to convert fat into fatty acids. Because of its breakdown process, protein will help you feel full longer. According to Susan Kleiner, PhD, RD, and the author of *Power Eating*, "Subjects placed on high-protein, moderate-carbohydrate meals had a greater and longer-lasting sensation of fullness compared with those on high-fat meals." Note that Dr. Kleiner cites *moderate* carbohydrate intake as the key.

JUST SAY NO TO FAT-FREE

The right kinds of fat, mono and polyunsaturated, are good for weight loss. Fat keeps us feeling physically full and emotionally satisfied—even though fat does not have as high a thermogenic effect as protein, it does trigger satiety mechanisms. Fat tastes good, which is psychologically satisfying. It's also physically satisfying, as it adds to the release of leptin, a hormone that signals the brain that the body is getting full. When you opt for a fat-free option, not only will you not feel as full, but you're also probably sacrificing a little fat for a lot of sugar. Some of the fat-free options have the same number of calories as the full-fat options, but because we assume fat-free means lower in calories, we eat more. Couple that with the fact that you are not feeling as physically full, and . . . do you see the train wreck just waiting to happen?

> **NOTE:** Always choose the low-fat option if it is available. One or two percent fat yogurt, cottage cheese, or milk should always be your first choice. However, it is important to know that even low-fat cheese (such as low-fat mozzarella) is still around 70 percent fat, so keep the portion limited to about an ounce per serving.

INCLUDE 1,200 MILLIGRAMS OF CALCIUM EACH DAY

According to a twenty-four-week case study conducted by Dr. Michael Zemel, director of the Nutrition Institute at the University of Tennessee, more calcium consumed translated into more weight loss. All the participants were on a diet that was 500 calories lower than their respective basal metabolic rates.

Here are the findings from the Zemel study:

• Group 1 consumed between 400 and 500 milligrams of calcium and lost 14.5 pounds.

- Group 2 consumed between 400 and 500 milligrams of calcium and a calcium supplement to increase their intake to 1,256 milligrams, and they lost 18.9 pounds.

- Group 3 increased their daily calcium intake to 1,137 milligrams by consuming more actual daily products and lost 24.4 pounds.

Now, I want to be very honest with you about this study and another one that also showed a direct relationship between dairy consumption and weight loss. One study was funded by the National Dairy Council and the other by General Mills, which makes Yoplait yogurt, and both have been the subject of a great deal of debate. I personally attended a seminar to listen to Dr. Zemel explain his study and findings, and I have to say that his argument was very compelling and his research appeared sound. I have also tested this theory on myself and many clients with great success. The reason behind the accelerated weight loss associated with dairy is that in the absence of calcium, the hormone calcitriol increases. According to Zemel, calcitriol "shuts off the mechanisms that break down fat and activates those that make it." Another research study reported in *Men's Health* suggests that dairy foods may help curb your appetite. The study showed that men who ate a low-fat diet that included dairy increased their levels of a satiating hormone, cholecys-tokinin, by about 20 percent. Finally, the Heritage Family Study, published in the *Journal of Nutrition*, "found an association between calcium intake and a reduction in body fat, especially abdominal fat, in men and white women."

If you can't consume the dairy because you are lactose intolerant or want to avoid dairy for some other reason, then eat sardines and calcium-rich fruits and vegetables. Or you can always opt for a calcium supplement, but it is important to note that the general rule of thumb pertaining to any supplement is that nutrient absorption by the body is about half of what it would be for a food containing the same nutrient. Your best sources of calcium are:

- one cup of skim, 1 percent, or 2 percent milk: *300 mg.*

- one cup of yogurt: *350 mg.*

- 1.5 ounces of cheddar cheese: *300 mg.*

- a half cup of broccoli, green beans, or sweet potato: *40 mg.*

- one cup cooked spinach: *250 mg.*

- one ounce of almonds: *75 mg.*

- one medium orange: *50 mg.*

- three ounces of sardines: *200 mg.*

CONSUME ONLY HIGH-FIBER CARBOHYDRATES

All carbs are *not* created equal. I want you to minimize, and ideally avoid, processed carbohydrates—white rice, pasta, bread, cookies, and cake— and instead, choose whole wheat, whole grains, unprocessed foods, fruits, and vegetables. Processed carbs, known as simple carbs, are considered high-glycemic foods, as they quickly turn to sugar when digested. The pancreas then releases insulin to pull the sugar out of your bloodstream and into your cells. Hopefully, it will be used for fuel rather than stored as fat. Once the sugar is swept out of your bloodstream, you are back to having low blood sugar, and you get hungry again. You can see how this vicious cycle occurs and is a recipe for certain weight gain. Even worse, when you continually consume high-glycemic foods, your pancreas is asked to repeatedly keep pumping out insulin, and, at some point, you overuse the system so much that it gets out of whack. Then the pancreas is ultimately unable to regulate all the sugar in your bloodstream. This higher level of sugar in your blood is also known as diabetes. Complex carbohydrates, such as most fruits and vegetables, legumes, and whole grain products, do not cause a spike in blood sugar. They contain more fiber, and fiber slows down digestion—this, in turn, maintains far more stable blood sugar levels.

Be careful when selecting certain foods boasting "healthy" carbs. Ever since the low-carb craze hit the market, food companies have scrambled to make it very difficult to successfully navigate your way through a grocery store. Don't be duped by brown-colored products that claim to be whole wheat, but might not be. Instead, read labels and look for "whole grain" or "whole wheat" at the top of the ingredient list. That's the only way to be 100 percent sure you are getting the real thing.

Like protein, complex carbohydrates help with satiety. According to Eric Rimm, associate professor of epidemiology and nutrition at the Harvard School of Public Health, the extra fiber in whole grains "leads to satiety and reduces the speed with which the meal is absorbed." Fiber makes you feel full, which means you eat less.

NOTE: It is important that you take on the challenge of avoiding simple carbs realistically, as they are enormously present in today's society. I don't want you to set yourself up to feel like a failure. We all are going to eat some white carbs from time to time. That's life, and this *is* America. You are going to eat birthday cake, some sushi, Thai, or Chinese food with white rice, and who can resist when your kids offer a taste of the cookie batter they are concocting just for you? Eat a bite or even a small portion, and then move on.

Here is a list of the high-fiber carbohydrates that are recommended on the Cardio-Free Diet:

Food	Serving Size	Fiber Content
Grains and Cereals		
Oatmeal	1 cup	4.0
Whole-wheat bread	1 slice	1.9
Whole-wheat spaghetti	1 cup	6.3
Brown rice	1 cup	2.0
All-Bran cereal	⅓ cup	8.5
Vegetables		
Spinach	1 cup	1.2
Broccoli	1 cup	4.4
Tomato	1 medium	1.5
Asparagus	1 cup	2.0
Green pepper	½ cup sliced	0.5
Baked potato with skin	1 medium	4.4
Fruits		
Apple with skin	1 medium	3.5
Orange	1 medium	2.6
Blueberries	1 cup	3.5
Pineapple	1 cup	2.2
Strawberries	1 cup	3.0
Legumes, Nuts, and Seeds		
Kidney beans	½ cup	7.3
Lima beans	½ cup	4.5
Lentils	½ cup	7.8
Almonds	10 nuts	1.1
Peanuts	10 nuts	1.4

ALWAYS SKIP LIQUID CALORIES

Liquid calories don't trigger satiety mechanisms. There was a case study that took one group of people and had them consume 450 calories of jelly beans each day. A second group was asked to consume 450 calories of liquid, such as juice, soda, or a sports drink. Both groups were told not to diet, but to record everything they ate. At the end of the study, the researchers found that the jelly bean eaters actually ate less—450 fewer calories a day, to be exact. Their bodies recognized the 450 calories in the jelly beans, but the liquid calorie group just kept eating, as if the liquid calories didn't register. Eat an orange and your body says, "I just had something to eat." Drink a glass of orange juice and your body asks, "Where's the food?" and keeps on eating. Plus, the juice is about 15 calories an ounce, so an eight-ounce glass is 120 calories. The average orange is only about 100 calories.

In this regard, Starbucks has really done a disservice to the American dieter. Did you know that the Double Chocolate Chip Frappuccino Blended Crème is 580 calories? Even the Caffè Mocha is 300 calories without whipped cream and 400 calories with it. Most people are drinking these concoctions every day, sometimes several times a day. There's nothing wrong with coffee. Regular or decaffeinated black coffee has between zero and 10 calories a cup. The problem lies in the cream, whole milk, whipped cream, caramel sauce, and whatever else they've dreamed up to add. Ditto with smoothies from places like Jamba Juice. Many of these drinks are 300, 400, 500 calories or more.

And a final note on almost everyone's favorite liquid calorie, alcohol. In Phase I of this eating plan, you should avoid alcohol altogether. In the subsequent phases, you can have a glass or two of wine. But, as with food, you must count the calories and realize that alcohol calories are dangerous, because they add up quickly. Here are a few examples. (Note: All caloric values are for one ounce.)

- white wine: *20–25 calories*, depending on the proof

- red wine: *20–25 calories*, but generally on the high end because of the proof

- gin, vodka, rum, and whiskey: 80 proof = *64 calories*; 90 proof = *73 calories*; 100 proof = *82 calories*

- sake: *39 calories*

- Baileys: *72 calories*

- Miller Lite: *8 calories*

- Guinness: *9.2 calories*

- FYI: A can of Red Bull has *113 calories*, and that is before you add alcohol to it!

NOTE: You must pay special attention to tropical drinks such as margaritas, piña coladas, or strawberry daiquiris, as they can easily get up over 400–500 calories per drink! These concoctions are especially dangerous, as they contain a large amount of juice and alcohol (double whammy), causing the calories to add up quickly, and most people don't stop at just one.

As a rule, always be a two-fisted drinker—consume two ounces of water for every ounce of alcohol. You won't drink as much that night, and you will thank me in the morning.

BE ON THE LOOKOUT FOR HIDDEN FAT

There is added or hidden fat in many of the most common foods, whether they are prepared at home or eaten out. Even boneless, skinless chicken breast is 25 percent fat. Some salmon can be as much as 50 percent fat. Low-fat dairy contains fat, as does all cheese and nuts. Therefore, I urge you to be very, very careful when consuming foods that contain high amounts of fat on this eating plan. That's why the portion sizes are so clear in the Cardio-Free Eating Plan. If you are not careful with the portions, then you are probably taking in more calories than you think.

BE CAUTIOUS WHEN ADDING FAT

While I do not add fat in the Cardio-Free Eating Plan, here are the items, in particular, that you must be careful with if you choose to include them after Phase IV:

- **cream** (*37 calories per tablespoon*) or **half and half** (*20 calories per tablespoon*) in your coffee

- **butter and margarine:** 100 calories per tablespoon. There are many lower-calorie, healthy alternatives to butter and margarine presently on the market.

- **olive oil:** It's 120 calories a tablespoon and pure fat (even though it's the good kind). Are you surprised to see that olive oil has *more* calories than either butter or margarine? If food is shining back at you, odds are it is covered with oil, frequently olive oil. Remember:

Shine and Glimmer Won't Make You Slimmer

- **salad dressing:** Don't be fooled by vinaigrette. It is three parts oil and one part vinegar, and many times it has the same calorie content as a creamy ranch or French dressing. Research has shown that as much as 15 percent of the average woman's daily caloric intake comes from salad dressing alone. Skip the dressing, and you could weigh a whole lot less next year. Opt for balsamic, raspberry, or red wine vinegar, lemon, or a dressing you make yourself using very little oil. Use spices freely—these help a great deal.

• **avocado:** It's the good fat, but a lot of it. An average avocado may be close to 400 calories.

• **dips:** If you didn't make it, odds are it is very high in calories and fat. Sour cream is 26 calories per tablespoon, and it is the base for most dips.

• **premium ice cream:** truly off the charts in fat and calories. A half cup of Ben & Jerry's Fudge Central is 300 calories. The pint is 1,200 calories. How many times have you eaten the whole container?

If you are going to consume any of these foods, then you must make sure that you are doing so in a portion-controlled manner. Because of the caloric density of these items, this is not really much food at all.

SIGNAL YOUR BODY WHEN IT IS TIME TO STOP EATING

Years ago, as an overweight child, I used to brush my teeth after eating as a way to signal my brain that it was time to stop. I still do that to this day. I also frequently chew gum when I am done eating. That way, if something catches my eye after breakfast, lunch, or dinner, but before my snack, the gum helps remind me that the eating is over. I'm a Chicago guy, so I love Wrigley's Extra, as it is sugar-free, only 5 calories a piece, and gives me the sensation of eating something sweet.

CHAPTER 11

The Cardio-Free Eating Plan

For women, the basis of the Cardio-Free Eating Plan is a 3-3-3 strategy. You will eat 300 calories each for breakfast, lunch, and dinner, as well as three 100-calorie snacks throughout the day. That will total 1,200 calories a day in Phase I.

For men, your program will be slightly higher in calories. You will also follow the 3-3-3 meal strategy, but your three snacks will contain 200 calories instead of the 100 for women. That means you will consume a total of 1,500 calories a day in Phase I.

Phase I lasts for the first two weeks. Then, as you enter Phases II, III, and IV, you will add an additional 100 calories to your diet each week by slightly increasing the portions of each meal, while keeping the caloric value of the snacks constant.

Turn the page to see how the diet will look in each phase.

Phase	Women	Calories	Men	Calories
I	Breakfast	300	Breakfast	300
	Snack	100	Snack	200
	Lunch	300	Lunch	300
	Snack	100	Snack	200
	Dinner	300	Dinner	300
	Snack	100	Snack	200
	Total	**1,200**	**Total**	**1,500**
II	Breakfast	333	Breakfast	333
	Snack	100	Snack	200
	Lunch	333	Lunch	333
	Snack	100	Snack	200
	Dinner	334	Dinner	334
	Snack	100	Snack	200
	Total	**1,300**	**Total**	**1,600**
III	Breakfast	366	Breakfast	366
	Snack	100	Snack	200
	Lunch	366	Lunch	366
	Snack	100	Snack	200
	Dinner	368	Dinner	368
	Snack	100	Snack	200
	Total	**1,400**	**Total**	**1,700**

Phase	Women	Calories	Men	Calories
IV	Breakfast	400	Breakfast	400
	Snack	100	Snack	200
	Lunch	400	Lunch	400
	Snack	100	Snack	200
	Dinner	400	Dinner	400
	Snack	100	Snack	200
	Total	**1,500**	**Total**	**1,800**

It is vital that you remain in your respective Phase IV caloric level until your have attained the weight you set out to achieve. In most cases, that may be the number of calories you will need to consume on an ongoing basis to maintain the loss. It is important to remember that weight loss and maintenance are not that far apart in terms of calories required. There are two reasons why this is the case:

1. Life will continually present opportunities to gain weight, whether it is the holidays, a family reunion, or crunch time at the office. Therefore, you will frequently find yourself back on the weight loss track to get those extra pounds off before they become a problem.

2. You will continue to age. While I want you to stall this process as much as possible, the truth is that weight gain gets easier as we age, due to a decrease in resting metabolism (even with the strength training, some diminishment is inevitable) and we move less, resulting in fewer calories expended through activity. Keeping your calories down will help minimize this risk.

I begin Phase I at 1,200 and 1,500 calories respectively, because in the beginning stages of a new plan, it is exciting to see dramatic results. In addition, you are most motivated and committed to making this plan work in the very beginning—and if you follow the Cardio-Free Eating and Exercise Plans, it will. In the first two weeks, you will notice a drastic change in how you look and feel. It is important to keep this momentum rolling as much as possible, because all the research and my professional experience indicate that after a while, we all start to cheat a little and eat more. The additional 100 calories added in each phase will help you fight that urge. When most people feel they are *off* the diet, they completely throw in the towel and revert to their old style of eating (which led to a higher body weight in the first place). By giving you the license to eat more during each phase, you will be more likely to stick with this plan for good.

THE CARDIO-FREE PHASE I AND II EATING PLAN

NOTE: Modifications for Phase III appear after each day's menu in Phase I; modifications for Phase IV appear after each day's menu in Phase II.

PHASE I: DAY 1

Breakfast: Sunrise Omelet

4 egg whites: *60 calories*
1 cup sliced tomatoes: *38 calories*
1 cup diced green peppers: *26 calories*
1 cup broccoli, cut into small florets: *24 calories*
½ ounces low-fat cheddar cheese, grated: *135 calories*
Cooking spray: *7 calories*
Salt and pepper to taste

Total: *290 calories*

Combine egg whites, veggies, cheese, salt, and pepper. Coat the inside of a nonstick skillet with cooking spray and turn heat to medium-high. Add the mixture. When the bottom side of the omelet is solid, flip or fold over with a spatula and cook the other side until done.

Snack (Women): ½ cup 2% cottage cheese: *90 calories*
Snack (Men): 1 cup 2% cottage cheese: *180 calories*

Lunch: Kiwi Shrimp Salad

1 large kiwi: *55 calories*
6 ounces cooked shrimp: *168 calories*
1 medium cucumber, sliced: *39 calories*
3 cups mixed greens: *24 calories*
2 tablespoons balsamic vinegar: *20 calories*
Salt and pepper to taste

Total: *306 calories*

Place cooked shrimp, sliced cucumber, and kiwi over the bed of mixed greens. Season and drizzle balsamic vinegar over the top.

Snack (Women): 12 almonds: *91 calories*
Snack (Men): 25 almonds: *190 calories*

Dinner: Grilled Chicken and Squash

4 ounces boneless, skinless chicken breast: *192 calories*
1 large zucchini: *62 calories*
1 medium yellow squash: *27 calories*
2 cups broccoli florets: *48 calories*
Dried basil and dried oregano to taste: *0 calories*
Salt and pepper to taste

Total: *329 calories*

Season chicken and veggies with basil, oregano, salt, and pepper. Place directly on grill and cook until veggies are tender and chicken is cooked through.

Snack (Women): 100-calorie low-fat yogurt
Snack (Men): 100-calorie low-fat yogurt and
1 cup sliced pineapple: *178 calories*

PHASE III: ADD THE FOLLOWING INGREDIENTS

Breakfast: 1 egg white (15 calories) and ½ ounce low-fat cheddar cheese (45 calories) = *60 additional calories*

Lunch: 2 ounces cooked shrimp (56 calories), 1 cup mixed greens (8 calories), and 1 tablespoon balsamic vinegar (10 calories) = *74 additional calories*

Dinner: 1 ounce chicken breast (48 calories) and ½ cup broccoli florets (12 calories) = *60 additional calories*

(Women Total) Phase I: 1,206 calories / Phase III: 1,400 calories
(Men Total) Phase I: 1,473 calories / Phase III: 1,667 calories

PHASE I: DAY 2

Breakfast: Poached Eggs

2 poached eggs: *180 calories*
100-calorie low-fat yogurt
½ slice of whole wheat toast: *40 calories*
Salt and pepper to taste

Total: *320 calories*

Poach eggs in three inches of barely simmering, acidulated water (use 1½ tablespoons of vinegar or 3 tablespoons of lemon juice) until the whites are set, about three minutes, and season with salt and pepper. Toast ½ slice of whole wheat toast, and dunk in yogurt if you like.

Snack (Women): 1 medium-size orange: *65 calories*
Snack (Men): 1 medium-size orange and
1 packet plain instant oatmeal: *165 calories*

Lunch: Grilled Chicken and Pear Salad

4 ounces boneless, skinless grilled chicken breast, sliced: *192 calories*
1 medium-size pear: *98 calories*
3 cups mixed greens: *24 calories*
2 tablespoons raspberry vinegar: *14 calories*
Salt and pepper to taste

Total: *328 calories*

Slice chicken and pears into strips and lay over bed of spinach leaves. Season and drizzle vinegar over the top.

Snack (Women): ½ cup 2% cottage cheese: *90 calories*
Snack (Men): 1 cup 2% cottage cheese: *180 calories*

Dinner: Lemon Swordfish

6 ounces swordfish: *264 calories*
1 cup broccoli florets: *24 calories*
½ cup parsley: *10 calories*
4 tablespoons lemon juice: *16 calories*
2 teaspoons water: *0 calories*
Salt and pepper to taste

Total: *314 calories*

Combine parsley, lemon juice, water, salt, and pepper, and spread over fish in baking pan. Bake in center of oven at 400 degrees for 12 to 15 minutes or until fish is fully cooked and flakes easily with a fork. Steam and serve broccoli on the side.

Snack (Women): 1 piece of string cheese: *80 calories*
Snack (Men): 2 pieces of string cheese: *160 calories*

PHASE III: ADD THE FOLLOWING INGREDIENTS

Breakfast: ½ slice of whole wheat toast (40 calories) and ½ cup strawberries (23 calories) = *63 additional calories*

Lunch: 1 ounce chicken breast (48 calories),
1 cup mixed greens (8 calories), and 1 tablespoon raspberry vinegar (7 calories) = *63 additional calories*

Dinner: 1 ounce swordfish (44 calories) and
1½ cups broccoli florets (36 calories) = *80 additional calories*

(Women Total) Phase I: 1,197 calories / Phase III: 1,403 calories
(Men Total) Phase I: 1,467 calories / Phase III: 1,673 calories

PHASE I: DAY 3

Breakfast: Feta Vegetable Omelet

4 egg whites: *60 calories*
1 cup sliced tomatoes: *38 calories*
1 ounce feta cheese: *74 calories*
1 cup chopped zucchini: *28 calories*
1 cup boiled and chopped broccoli: *44 calories*

1 cup boiled and chopped spinach: *42 calories*
Cooking spray: *7 calories*

Total: *293 calories*

Coat the inside of a nonstick skillet with cooking spray. Combine all ingredients, add to the skillet, and cook over medium heat until the bottom of the omelet is solid. Then flip or fold over with a spatula and cook until done.

Snack (Women): 1 cup blueberries: *82 calories*
Snack (Men): 1 cup blueberries, 1 cup pineapple: *160 calories*

Lunch: Mixed Greens Ranch Salad

3 cups mixed greens: *24 calories*
1 cup sliced red pepper: *26 calories*
1 cup sliced green pepper: *26 calories*
½ cup chopped tomato: *19 calories*
1 cup sliced mushrooms: *18 calories*
¼ cup chickpeas: *67 calories*
2 tablespoons fat-free ranch dressing
   (there isn't a 1% or 2% option): *48 calories*
½ cup 2% cottage cheese: *90 calories*
Salt and pepper to taste

Total: *318 calories*

Combine lettuce, peppers, tomatoes, mushrooms, and chickpeas, and season. Mix fat-free ranch dressing with the cottage cheese and pour over salad.

Snack (Women): 100-calorie low-fat yogurt
Snack (Men): 100-calorie low-fat yogurt and ⅓ cup raisins: *208 calories*

Dinner: Apple Balsamic Chicken

4 ounces boneless, skinless chicken breast: *192 calories*
¾ cup diced apple: *48 calories*
¾ cup diced cranberries: *41 calories*
4 tablespoons balsamic vinegar: *40 calories*
Salt and pepper to taste

Total: *321 calories*

Preheat oven to 375 degrees. Place apples and cranberries over chicken in a baking dish. Season, top with balsamic vinegar, and bake until chicken is done and opaque throughout.

Snack (Women): ¼ cup roasted peanuts: *107 calories*
Snack (Men): ½ cup roasted peanuts: *214 calories*

PHASE III: ADD THE FOLLOWING INGREDIENTS

Breakfast: 1 egg white (15 calories) and ½ ounce feta (37 calories) = *52 additional calories*

Lunch: 1 cup mixed greens (8 calories), ½ cup red pepper (13 calories), ½ cup green pepper (13 calories), ½ cup mushrooms (9 calories), and 1 tablespoon fat-free ranch (24 calories) = *67 additional calories*

Dinner: 1 ounce of chicken breast (48 calories), ¼ cup sliced apple (16 calories), and ¼ cup cranberries (14 calories) = *78 additional calories*

(Women Total) Phase I: 1,221 calories / Phase III: 1,418 calories
(Men Total) Phase I: 1,514 calories / Phase III: 1,711 calories

PHASE I: DAY 4

Breakfast: Apple Banana Crunch

1½ cups diced apple: *96 calories*
1 container nonfat or low-fat banana yogurt: *100 calories*
1 cup Wheaties: *110 calories*

Total: *306 calories*

Warm apples if desired, or just combine ingredients in bowl or large glass and serve.

Snack (Women): ½ cup 2% cottage cheese: *90 calories*
Snack (Men): 1 cup 2% cottage cheese: *180 calories*

Lunch: Turkey Burger and Tomato

6 ounces low-fat (99% fat-free if possible) ground turkey: *285 calories*
1 medium-size tomato, sliced: *26 calories*
Cooking spray: *7 calories*
Salt and pepper to taste

Total: *318 calories*

Coat the inside of a pan with cooking spray. Season turkey, form into a patty, and cook over medium heat until cooked through. Top with a small amount of ketchup or mustard, if desired.

Snack (Women): 2 Reduced-Fat Wheat Thins crackers and
1 tablespoon peanut butter: *120 calories*
Snack (Men): 4 Reduced-Fat Wheat Thins crackers and
2 tablespoons peanut butter: *240 calories*

Dinner: Grilled Salmon

6 ounces salmon: *240 calories*
16 asparagus spears: *64 calories*
Salt and pepper to taste

Total: 304 calories

Season and grill salmon until it flakes easily with a fork, about 8 minutes per side. Season and grill asparagus until tender-crisp, about eight minutes, and sprinkle with lemon pepper seasoning if desired.

Snack (Women): 1 piece of string cheese: *80 calories*
Snack (Men): 1 piece of string cheese and ½ cup frozen shelled edamame, boiled in water for five minutes, then drained: *180 calories*

PHASE III: ADD THE FOLLOWING INGREDIENTS

Breakfast: ½ cup Wheaties = *55 additional calories*

Lunch: 1 ounce low-fat ground turkey (48 calories) and 3 pickle spears (12 calories) = *60 additional calories*

Dinner: 1 ounce salmon (40 calories) and 4 asparagus spears (16 calories) = *55 additional calories*

(Women Total) Phase I: 1,218 calories / Phase III: 1, 389 calories
(Men Total) Phase I: 1,528 calories / Phase III: 1,699 calories

PHASE I: DAY 5

Breakfast: Wheaties and Strawberries

1 cup Wheaties cereal: *110 calories*
1 cup 1% milk: *100 calories*
2 cups sliced strawberries: *92 calories*

Total: 302 calories

Top the cereal with strawberries and serve.

Snack (Women): 1 piece of string cheese: *80 calories*
Snack (Men): 1 piece of string cheese and 1 medium-size apple: *167 calories*

Lunch: Chicken Fajita

3 ounces boneless, skinless chicken breast: *144 calories*
1 cup sliced green pepper: *26 calories*
3 ounces tomato juice: *16 calories*
1 teaspoon chili powder: *8 calories*
1 teaspoon garlic powder: *10 calories*
2 corn tortillas: *120 calories*
Cooking spray: *7 calories*
Salt and pepper to taste

Total: *331 calories*

Coat the inside of a large skillet with cooking spray. Combine chicken, peppers, tomato juice, chili powder, garlic powder, salt, and pepper. Add to the pan and cook over medium-high heat until chicken is cooked through. Put mixture into warmed tortillas and serve.

Snack (Women): ¼ cup roasted peanuts: *107 calories*
Snack (Men): ½ cup roasted peanuts: *214 calories*

Dinner: Baked Whitefish

5 ounces whitefish fillet: *190 calories*
4 tablespoons lemon juice: *16 calories*
2 cloves garlic: *8 calories*
1 cup chopped carrots: *48 calories*

2 cups broccoli florets: *48 calories*

2 tablespoons water: *0 calories*

Total: *310 calories*

Preheat oven to 400 degrees. In a baking dish, combine water, carrots, lemon juice, and ¼ clove garlic. Sprinkle fish on both sides with salt and pepper to taste and rub remaining garlic all over. Push carrots to sides of the dish and lay fish on bottom. Bake about 45 minutes, stirring carrots every 15 minutes, until fish is golden and carrots are tender. Steam broccoli and serve separately.

Snack (Women): 100-calorie low-fat yogurt
Snack (Men): 100-calorie low-fat yogurt and
1 medium banana: *205 calories*

PHASE III: ADD THE FOLLOWING INGREDIENTS

Breakfast: ½ cup Wheaties = *55 additional calories*

Lunch: 1 ounce chicken breast (48 calories) and
½ cup diced tomato (19 calories) = *67 additional calories*

Dinner: 1 ounce whitefish (38 calories) and
½ cup chopped carrots (24 calories) = *62 additional calories*

(Women Total) Phase I: 1,230 calories / Phase III: 1,414 calories
(Men Total) Phase I: 1,529 calories / Phase III: 1,713 calories

PHASE I: DAY 6

Breakfast: Fruity Yogurt Delight

1 container low-fat vanilla yogurt: *100 calories*

1 cup blueberries: *82 calories*

1 cup raspberries: *62 calories*
1 cup sliced strawberries: *46 calories*

Total: *290 calories*

Combine all ingredients and serve.

Snack (Women): 1 Laughing Cow Light Garlic & Herb cheese wedge and 3 Reduced-Fat Triscuits: *107 calories*
Snack (Men): 2 Laughing Cow Light Garlic & Herb cheese wedges and 6 Reduced-Fat Triscuits: *214 calories*

Lunch: Whole Wheat Turkey Sandwich

2 slices whole wheat bread: *160 calories*
4 slices low-fat turkey: *46 calories*
2 pieces romaine lettuce: *2 calories*
2 tomato slices: *5 calories*
1 tablespoon spicy mustard: *4 calories*
1 medium pear: *98 calories*

Total: *315 calories*

Slice the pear and serve alongside the sandwich.

Snack (Women): 1 large hard-boiled egg: *90 calories*
Snack (Men): 2 large hard-boiled eggs: *180 calories*

Dinner: Chicken Kabobs

4 ounces boneless, skinless chicken breast: *192 calories*
2 cups whole mushrooms: *34 calories*
2 green peppers: *40 calories*
1 cup cherry tomatoes: *31 calories*

1 cup sliced zucchini: *28 calories*
Salt and pepper to taste

Total: *325 calories*

Cut seeded peppers and chicken into one-inch pieces. Place on skewers (soak for 30 minutes first if wood), alternating with mushrooms, tomatoes, and zucchini. Season and grill until chicken is cooked through.

Snack (Women): ½ cup 2% cottage cheese: *90 calories*
Snack (Men): 1 cup 2% cottage cheese: *180 calories*

PHASE III: ADD THE FOLLOWING INGREDIENTS

Breakfast: 1 slice whole wheat toast = *80 additional calories*

Lunch: 3 slices of low-fat turkey (34 calories) and 2 pickle spears (8 calories) = *42 additional calories*

Dinner: 1 ounce chicken breast (48 calories) and 1 cup sliced zucchini (28 calories) = *76 additional calories*

(Women Total) Phase I: 1,217 calories / Phase III: 1,415 calories
(Men Total) Phase I: 1,504 calories / Phase III: 1,702 calories

PHASE I: DAY 7

Breakfast: Creamy Eggs with Spinach and Tomato

5 egg whites: *75 calories*
2 cups chopped spinach: *24 calories*
1 cup diced tomatoes: *38 calories*
1 slice whole wheat toast: *80 calories*

½ cup 2% cottage cheese: *90 calories*
Cooking spray: *7 calories*

Total: *314 calories*

Combine egg whites, cottage cheese, spinach, and tomatoes. Coat the inside of a nonstick skillet with cooking spray. Add mixture to the skillet and cook over medium-high heat until done. Serve with toast.

Snack (Women): 12 almonds: *91 calories*
Snack (Men): 25 almonds: *190 calories*

Lunch: Turkey Chili

3 ounces low-fat ground turkey: *180 calories*
½ cup kidney beans: *27 calories*
4 ounces crushed tomatoes: *25 calories*
½ teaspoon chili powder: *4 calories*
¾ cup chopped green peppers: *20 calories*
¼ cup chopped onions: *15 calories*
1 teaspoon garlic powder: *12 calories*
Cooking spray: *7 calories*
⅛ cup water: *0 calories*
Salt and pepper to taste

Total: *290 calories*

In a nonstick skillet coated with cooking spray, combine green peppers, onions, and garlic powder. Cook over low heat until tender. Then add beans, tomatoes, water, turkey, and chili powder. Simmer for 25 minutes, season, and serve.

Snack (Women): ½ cup 2% cottage cheese and
1 stalk celery: *96 calories*
Snack (Men): 1 cup 2% cottage cheese and
2 stalks celery: *192 calories*

Dinner: Tuna Steak

5 ounces tuna steak: *205 calories*

1 lime: *20 calories*

2 tablespoons fresh parsley: *0 calories*

1 cup broccoli florets: *24 calories*

1 cup chopped carrots: *48 calories*

Black pepper to taste

Total: *297 calories*

Cut lime into thirds. Squeeze ⅔ lime and place 1 tablespoon finely chopped parsley onto nine-inch dish. Turn tuna in dish until it is covered in lime and let marinate in fridge for 30 minutes. Place tuna on boiling rack or on the grill and cook until pale pink in the center. Steam broccoli and carrots separately.

Snack (Women): 100-calorie low-fat yogurt
Snack (Men): 100-calorie low-fat yogurt and
1½ cups honeydew melon: *190 calories*

PHASE III: ADD THE FOLLOWING INGREDIENTS

Breakfast: 1 slice whole wheat toast = *80 additional calories*

Lunch: 1 ounce lean turkey = *60 additional calories*

Dinner: 1 ounce tuna steak (41 calories) and
1 cup broccoli florets (24 calories) = *65 additional calories*

(Women Total) Phase I: 1,188 calories / Phase III: 1,393 calories
(Men Total) Phase I: 1,473 calories / Phase III: 1,678 calories

PHASE I: DAY 8

Breakfast: Peanut Butter and Banana Oatmeal

1 packet plain instant oatmeal: *103 calories*
1 medium banana: *105 calories*
1 tablespoon peanut butter: *95 calories*

Total: *303 calories*

Mix oatmeal, peanut butter, and bananas and microwave as directed on package.

Snack (Women): ½ cup raw baby carrots and ½ cup 2% cottage cheese: *114 calories*
Snack (Men): 1 cup raw baby carrots and 1 cup 2% cottage cheese: *228 calories*

Lunch: Egg and Tuna Salad

3 ounces canned tuna in water, drained: *90 calories*
3 cups mixed greens: *24 calories*
20 medium seedless grapes: *30 calories*
1 cup chopped green peppers: *26 calories*
2 hard-boiled eggs (whites only), chopped: *30 calories*
½ cup 2% low-fat cottage cheese: *90 calories*
Salt and pepper to taste

Total: *290 calories*

Place lettuce in a bowl. Put cottage cheese and tuna on bed of lettuce. Add egg whites, green peppers, and red grapes.

Snack (Women): 1 piece of string cheese: *90 calories*
Snack (Men): 2 pieces of string cheese: *180 calories*

Dinner: Roast Turkey with Steamed Broccoli

1 cup white meat roast turkey (lean): *209 calories*
2 cups broccoli florets: *48 calories*
1 cup carrots: *48 calories*
Salt and pepper to taste

Total: *305 calories*

Place turkey in baking pan and cook at 350 degrees for 15 to 20 minutes until opaque or thoroughly cooked. Steam broccoli and carrots separately.

Snack (Women): 100-calorie low-fat yogurt
Snack (Men): 100-calorie low-fat yogurt and
2 sliced kiwis: *192 calories*

PHASE III: ADD THE FOLLOWING INGREDIENTS

Breakfast: 1 slice of whole wheat toast = *80 additional calories*

Lunch: 1 cup green peppers (26 calories) and 2 egg whites of boiled eggs (34 calories) = *60 additional calories*

Dinner: 1 cup carrots = *48 additional calories*

(Women Total) Phase I: 1,202 calories / Phase III: 1,390 calories
(Men Total) Phase I: 1,498 calories / Phase III: 1,686 calories

PHASE I: DAY 9

Breakfast: Fruit with Yogurt Dressing

1 container low-fat lemon yogurt: *100 calories*
1 cup sliced strawberries: *46 calories*
1 cup blueberries: *82 calories*
1 cup diced honeydew melon: *60 calories*

Total: *288 calories*

Combine fruit, top with lemon yogurt, and serve.

Snack (Women): 2 graham cracker squares with
2 teaspoons of peanut butter: *98 calories*
Snack (Men): 4 graham cracker squares with
4 teaspoons of peanut butter: *196 calories*

Lunch: Grilled Chicken Salad

4 cups mixed greens: *32 calories*
4 ounces grilled boneless, skinless chicken breast: *192 calories*
1 cup sliced green peppers: *26 calories*
1 cup sliced tomatoes: *38 calories*
2 tablespoons balsamic vinegar: *20 calories*

Total: *308 calories*

Combine the chicken with the vegetables, season, and drizzle with balsamic vinegar.

Snack (Women): 1 piece of string cheese: *80 calories*
Snack (Men): 1 piece of string cheese and
½ cup edamame: *180 calories*

Dinner: Ginger Fillet

6 ounces haddock fillet: *150 calories*

2 teaspoon ginger: *6 calories*

2 tablespoons ground basil: *22 calories*

2 cups broccoli florets: *48 calories*

2 cups chopped carrots: *48 calories*

Cooking spray: *7 calories*

Total: *281 calories*

Heat a nonstick twelve-inch skillet coated with cooking spray on medium-high until hot. Coat the fish with ginger and fresh basil, season with salt and pepper. Add to the skillet and cook until flounder is opaque and cooked through, about 5 minutes per side.

Snack (Women): ½ cup 2% cottage cheese and 1 medium tomato, sliced: *116 calories*
Snack (Men): 1 cup 2% cottage cheese and 1 medium tomato, sliced: *206 calories*

PHASE III: ADD THE FOLLOWING INGREDIENTS

Breakfast: 1 slice whole wheat toast = *80 additional calories*

Lunch: 1 ounce chicken breast (48 calories) and 1 tablespoon balsamic vinegar (10 calories) = *58 additional calories*

Dinner: 3 ounces haddock fillet = *75 additional calories*

(Women Total) Phase I: 1,171 calories / Phase III: 1,384 calories
(Men Total) Phase I: 1,459 calories / Phase III: 1,672 calories

PHASE I: DAY 10

Breakfast: Cranberry Crunch

1 cup 2% cottage cheese: *180 calories*
20 pieces dried cranberries: *21 calories*
10 almonds: *76 calories*

Total: 277 calories

Combine and serve.

Snack (Women): 100-calorie low-fat yogurt
Snack (Men): 100-calorie low-fat yogurt and
1 medium banana: *205 calories*

Lunch: Shrimp and Tomato Salad

4 ounces cooked shrimp: *112 calories*
1 ounce feta cheese: *74 calories*
1 medium cucumber, seeded and cubed: *39 calories*
2 cups Roma tomatoes, cubed: *76 calories*
2 tablespoons balsamic vinegar: *20 calories*
2 sprigs fresh parsley (leaves only): *0 calories*

Total: *321 calories*

*Combine cooked shrimp, cucumber, and tomatoes in a bowl. Sprinkle
with feta cheese, drizzle with balsamic vinegar, and sprinkle parsley
on top.*

Snack (Women): 1 medium-size apple: *87 calories*
Snack (Men): 1 medium-size apple and
1 tablespoon peanut butter: *182 calories*

Dinner: Pork Kabobs

4 ounces lean pork chop: *165 calories*
1 green bell pepper: *20 calories*
1 yellow bell pepper: *20 calories*
2 cups whole mushrooms: *36 calories*
2 cups cherry tomatoes: *62 calories*
Salt and pepper to taste

Total: *303 calories*

Cut pork chop and bell peppers into one-inch pieces. Alternate ingredients on skewers (if wood, soak in water for 30 minutes first) and grill until pork is cooked through.

Snack (Women): ½ cup baby raw carrots and
½ cup 2% cottage cheese: *114 calories*
Snack (Men): 1 cup baby raw carrots and
1 cup 2% cottage cheese: *228 calories*

PHASE III: ADD THE FOLLOWING INGREDIENTS

Breakfast: 1 slice whole wheat toast = *80 additional calories*

Lunch: 2 ounces cooked shrimp = *56 additional calories*

Dinner: 2 ounces lean pork = *83 additional calories*

(Women Total) Phase I: 1,202 calories / Phase III: 1,421 calories
(Men Total) Phase I: 1,516 calories / Phase III: 1,735 calories

PHASE I: DAY 11

Breakfast: Creamy Apple Cinnamon Oatmeal

1 packet plain instant oatmeal: *103 calories*
½ cup 1% milk: *50 calories*

1 cup sliced apples: *64 calories*

1 slice whole wheat toast: *80 calories*

2 teaspoons cinnamon: *12 calories*

Total: *309 calories*

Mix oatmeal, milk, and apple and microwave as directed. Top with cinnamon and serve.

Snack (Women): ½ cup 2% cottage cheese and ½ cup strawberries: *113 calories*

Snack (Men): 1 cup 2% cottage cheese and ½ cup strawberries: *203 calories*

Lunch: Stuffed Bell Pepper

1 bell pepper: *20 calories*

4 ounces ground lean turkey: *240 calories*

2 tablespoons chopped onion: *8 calories*

1 teaspoon crushed garlic: *5 calories*

1 tablespoon tomato paste: *13 calories*

1 teaspoon basil: *4 calories*

Salt and pepper to taste

Total: *290 calories*

Preheat oven to 375 degrees. Cut off the top of the bell pepper, then reach in to remove the seeds and core. Separately, combine turkey, onions, garlic, basil, salt, and pepper. Stuff the bell pepper with the filling and spread tomato paste thinly over the top. Place on cookie sheet and bake in oven for 30 minutes or until turkey is cooked completely.

Snack (Women): 10 cashew nuts: *91 calories*

Snack (Men): 20 cashew nuts: *182 calories*

Dinner: Herbed Chicken and Grilled Veggies

4 ounces boneless, skinless chicken breast: *192 calories*

½ clove garlic, finely chopped: *2 calories*

¼ tablespoon rosemary: *0 calories*

¼ tablespoon thyme: *0 calories*

2 tablespoons dry white wine: *19 calories*

1 large zucchini: *62 calories*

1 cup broccoli florets: *24 calories*

Salt and pepper to taste

Total: *299 calories*

Make a marinade by combining garlic, herbs, and wine in a small bowl. Reserve a little marinade for the veggies, and coat the chicken with the rest. Marinate in the refrigerator for two hours. Season chicken with salt and pepper and grill until cooked through. Season and grill the whole veggies until tender-crisp. Brush reserved marinade on veggies.

Snack (Women): 1 piece of string cheese: *80 calories*
Snack (Men): 2 pieces of string cheese: *160 calories*

PHASE III: ADD THE FOLLOWING INGREDIENTS

Breakfast: 1 cup sliced apple = *64 additional calories*

Lunch: 1 ounce lean turkey = *60 additional calories*

Dinner: 1 ounce chicken breast (48 calories) and
1 cup broccoli florets (24 calories) = *72 additional calories*

(Women Total) Phase I: 1,182 calories / Phase III: 1,378 calories
(Men Total) Phase I: 1,443 calories / Phase III: 1,639 calories

PHASE I: DAY 12

Breakfast: Nectarine Apricot Yogurt

1 cup low-fat vanilla yogurt: *100 calories*
1 cup nectarine, sliced: *68 calories*
1 cup apricot, sliced: *74 calories*
½ cup pineapple: *39 calories*

Total: *281 calories*

Combine and serve.

Snack (Women): 3 pieces of rolled-up low-fat
turkey breast with half of a tomato and 1 tablespoon
Dijon mustard: *97 calories*
Snack (Men): 6 pieces of rolled-up low-fat turkey
breast with one tomato and 2 tablespoons Dijon
mustard: *194 calories*

Lunch: Mixed Green Salad with Fruit and Nuts

3 cups mixed greens: *24 calories*
1 cup mandarin orange: *86 calories*
1 cup sliced apple: *64 calories*
¼ cup roasted peanuts: *107 calories*
½ cup raspberries: *31 calories*

Total: *312 calories*

*Place mixed greens in large bowl, top with fruits, sprinkle with peanuts,
and serve.*

Snack (Women): 100-calorie low-fat yogurt
Snack (Men): 100-calorie low-fat yogurt and
⅓ cup raisins: *208 calories*

Dinner: Tomato Artichoke Chicken

4 ounces grilled boneless, skinless chicken breast: *192 calories*

1 cup diced tomato: *38 calories*

½ cup diced green pepper: *13 calories*

½ cup marinara sauce: *37 calories*

½ cup artichoke hearts: *42 calories*

Salt and pepper to taste

Total: *322 calories*

Grill chicken. In large saucepan, combine green pepper, marinara sauce, tomatoes, and artichokes. Simmer over a low heat for 10 to 15 minutes or until green peppers have softened. Adjust seasoning if needed, pour mixture over chicken, and serve.

Snack (Women): 1 piece of string cheese: *80 calories*
Snack (Men): 2 pieces of string cheese: *160 calories*

PHASE III: ADD THE FOLLOWING INGREDIENTS

Breakfast: 1 slice of whole wheat toast = *80 additional calories*

Lunch: ¼ cup roasted peanuts = *54 additional calories*

Dinner: 1 ounce chicken breast (48 calories) and
8 asparagus spears (32 calories) = *78 additional calories*

(Women Total) Phase I: 1,192 calories / Phase III: 1,406 calories
(Men Total) Phase I: 1,477 calories / Phase III: 1,691 calories

PHASE I: DAY 13

Breakfast: Berry Yogurt

1 cup low-fat vanilla yogurt: *100 calories*

1 cup sliced nectarine: *68 calories*

1 cup blueberries: *82 calories*

1 cup sliced strawberries: *46 calories*

Total: *296 calories*

Combine fruit, top with vanilla yogurt, and serve.

Snack (Women): Hard-boiled egg: *90 calories*
Snack (Men): 2 hard-boiled eggs: *180 calories*

Lunch: Grilled Chicken and Steamed Veggies

4 ounces grilled boneless, skinless chicken breast: *192 calories*

1 large zucchini: *62 calories*

1½ cups broccoli florets: *36 calories*

1 medium yellow squash: *27 calories*

1 teaspoon basil: *4 calories*

1 teaspoon oregano: *6 calories*

Salt and pepper to taste

Total: *327 calories*

Steam the vegetables until tender-crisp and season. Serve with chicken and top everything with basil and oregano.

Snack (Women): 1 grapefruit: *92 calories*
Snack (Men): 1 grapefruit and 10 cashews: *183 calories*

Dinner: Broiled Cod Fillet

4 ounces broiled cod fillet: *120 calories*

2 teaspoons ginger: *12 calories*

2 tablespoons ground basil: *22 calories*

2 cups broccoli: *48 calories*

1 cup fresh green beans: *34 calories*
1 ounce low-fat cheddar cheese: *90 calories*
Salt and pepper to taste

Total: *326 calories*

Sprinkle basil and ginger over cod fillet. Season and broil fish until thoroughly cooked. Next, steam veggies for side dish. Melt cheddar over broccoli.

Snack (Women): ½ cup 2% cottage cheese: *90 calories*
Snack (Men): 1 cup 2% cottage cheese: *180 calories*

PHASE III: ADD THE FOLLOWING INGREDIENTS

Breakfast: 1 slice whole wheat toast (80 calories) = *80 additional calories*

Lunch: 1 ounce chicken breast (48 calories) and ½ cup broccoli florets (12 calories) = *60 additional calories*

Dinner: Add 2 ounces cod fillet = *60 additional calories*

(Women Total) Phase I: 1,221 calories / Phase III: 1,421 calories
(Men Total) Phase I: 1,492 calories / Phase III: 1,692 calories

PHASE I: DAY 14

Breakfast: Broccoli Cheese Omelet

4 egg whites: *60 calories*
2 cups broccoli, cut into small florets: *48 calories*
2 slices low-fat American cheese: *62 calories*

1 slice whole wheat toast: *80 calories*

2 teaspoons of jam: *35 calories*

Cooking spray: *7 calories*

Salt and pepper to taste

Total: *292 calories*

Combine broccoli and cheese with egg whites. Coat the inside of a non-stick skillet with cooking spray, and cook mixture over medium heat. When the bottom side of the omelet is solid, flip or fold with a spatula and cook the other side. Serve with toast and jam.

Snack (Women): 100-calorie low-fat yogurt

Snack (Men): 100-calorie low-fat yogurt, 1 cup nectarine, and 1 cup strawberries: *214 calories*

Lunch: Whole Wheat Wrap

1 eight-inch whole wheat tortilla wrap: *159 calories*

½ cup diced cucumber: *7 calories*

½ cup romaine lettuce: *4 calories*

½ cup chopped tomato: *19 calories*

3 tablespoons fat-free ranch dressing: *72 calories*

1 cup sprouts: *30 calories*

Total: *291 calories*

On one half of the tortilla, combine lettuce, cucumbers, and tomatoes, and top with fat-free ranch dressing and roll up.

Snack (Women): 1 piece of string cheese: *80 calories*

Snack (Men): 2 pieces of string cheese: *160 calories*

Dinner: Creamy Mushroom Turkey

1 cup white meat roast turkey (lean): *209 calories*
½ cup low-fat cream of mushroom soup: *65 calories*
1 cup fresh green beans: *34 calories*

Total: *308 calories*

Place turkey in baking pan and smother with cream of mushroom soup. Cook at 350 degrees for 15 to 20 minutes until opaque or thoroughly cooked. Steam side of green beans separately.

Snack (Women): 12 almonds: *91 calories*
Snack (Men): 25 almonds: *190 calories*

PHASE III: ADD THE FOLLOWING INGREDIENTS

Breakfast: 2 egg whites (30 calories) and 1 slice low-fat American cheese (31 calories) = *61 additional calories*

Lunch: 1 apple = *87 additional calories*

Dinner: 1 cup green beans (34 calories) and 1 cup chopped carrots (48 calories) = *82 additional calories*

(Women Total) Phase I: 1,162 calories / Phase III: 1,392 calories
(Men Total) Phase I: 1,455 calories / Phase III: 1,685 calories

PHASE II: DAY 15

Breakfast: Cottage Cheese and Toast

½ cup 2% low-fat cottage cheese: *90 calories*
2 slices whole wheat bread: *160 calories*
2 teaspoons all-fruit spread: *36 calories*
¾ cup sliced apple: *48 calories*

Total: *334 calories*

Mix chopped apples with cottage cheese. Toast wheat bread and spread fruit spread on top.

Snack (Women): 12 almonds: *91 calories*
Snack (Men): 25 almonds: *190 calories*

Lunch: Tuna Veggie Salad

3 ounces canned tuna in water, drained: *90 calories*

3 cups spinach leaves: *24 calories*

½ cup chopped tomatoes: *19 calories*

1 medium cucumber, sliced: *39 calories*

1 cup sliced green pepper: *26 calories*

2 tablespoons fat-free ranch dressing: *48 calories*

12 almonds: *91 calories*

Total: *337 calories*

Put spinach into large bowl. Add tomatoes, cucumber, green pepper, and almonds. Add tuna and drizzle with fat-free ranch dressing.

Snack (Women): 1½ cups raspberries: *93 calories*
Snack (Men): 1½ cups raspberries and
1½ cups blueberries: *216 calories*

Dinner: Chicken Tacos

2 ounces boneless, skinless chicken breast: *96 calories*

½ cup shredded red cabbage: *10 calories*

2 corn tortillas: *90 calories*

½ cup red onion: *30 calories*

2 tablespoons salsa: *12 calories*

1 ounce low-fat shredded cheddar cheese: *90 calories*

Total: *328 calories*

Place chicken on grill until thoroughly cooked, then add all other ingredients in corn tortillas.

Snack (Women): 100-calorie low-fat yogurt
Snack (Men): 100-calorie low-fat yogurt and
1 cup sliced pineapple: *178 calories*

PHASE IV: ADD THE FOLLOWING INGREDIENTS

Breakfast: 1¼ cups sliced apples = *80 additional calories*

Lunch: 1 ounce canned tuna (30 calories),
1 cup spinach (8 calories), and 1 tablespoon fat-free ranch dressing
(24 calories) = *62 additional calories*

Dinner: 1 ounce chicken breast (48 calories) and 1 tablespoon salsa
(6 calories) = *54 additional calories*

(Women Total) Phase II: 1,283 calories / Phase IV: 1,479 calories
(Men Total) Phase II: 1,583 calories / Phase IV: 1,779 calories

PHASE II: DAY 16

Breakfast: Poached Eggs

2 eggs: *180 calories*
100-calorie low-fat yogurt
1½ cups sliced strawberries: *69 calories*
Salt and pepper to taste

Total: *349 calories*

Poach 2 eggs in three inches of barely simmering, acidulated water (use 1½ tablespoons of vinegar or 3 tablespoons of lemon juice) until the whites are set, about 3 minutes, and season with salt and pepper. Mix strawberries with yogurt.

Snack (Women): 1 piece of string cheese: *80 calories*
Snack (Men): 2 pieces of string cheese: *160 calories*

Lunch: Veggie Burger

1 veggie burger: *150 calories*
1 slice whole wheat bread: *80 calories*
1 medium-size tomato, sliced: *26 calories*
1 tablespoon each, ketchup and mustard: *21 calories*
3 pickle spears: *12 calories*
½ cup baby carrots: *24 calories*

Total: *313 calories*

Cook burger per package instructions, and top with tomato, lettuce, ketchup, and mustard. Serve with pickles and carrots.

Snack (Women): 12 almonds: *91 calories*
Snack (Men): 25 almonds: *190 calories*

Dinner: Chicken Cacciatore

4 ounces boneless, skinless chicken breast: *192 calories*
1 tablespoon chopped onion: *4 calories*
½ clove chopped garlic: *2 calories*
1 cup chopped green pepper: *26 calories*
1 cup whole peeled tomato: *25 calories*
1 cup fresh green beans: *34 calories*
1 cup chopped carrots: *48 calories*
⅛ teaspoon oregano: *0 calories*
Cooking spray: *7 calories*

Total: *338 calories*

Coat a large nonstick skillet with cooking spray and sauté onion and garlic over medium heat until soft. Add chicken. Stir in tomatoes, oregano, and beans. Reduce heat to medium low and simmer for 8 to 10 minutes, stirring occasionally. Steam carrots for side dish. Remove chicken from heat and serve.

Snack (Women): ½ cup 2% cottage cheese and 2 fresh peach slices: *109 calories*
Snack (Men): 1 cup 2% cottage cheese and 2 fresh peach slices: *199 calories*

PHASE IV: ADD THE FOLLOWING INGREDIENTS

Breakfast: 1 slice whole wheat toast = *80 additional calories*

Lunch: 2 tablespoons each, ketchup and mustard (21 calories), and ½ cup carrots (24 calories) = *45 additional calories*

Dinner: 1 ounce chicken breast (48 calories) and 1 cup green beans (34 calories) = *82 additional calories*

(Women Total) Phase II: 1,280 calories / Phase IV: 1,487 calories
(Men Total) Phase II: 1,549 calories / Phase IV: 1,756 calories

PHASE II: DAY 17

Breakfast: Berry Oatmeal

1 packet plain instant oatmeal: *103 calories*
1 cup blueberries: *82 calories*
1 cup sliced strawberries: *46 calories*
½ cup raspberries: *31 calories*
½ cup 1% milk: *50 calories*

Total: *312 calories*

Mix oatmeal and milk and microwave for 45 seconds on high. Stir in berries and microwave for 15 seconds.

Snack (Women): 10 cashew nuts: *91 calories*
Snack (Men): 20 cashew nuts: *182 calories*

Lunch: Tuna Melt

3 ounces canned tuna in water, drained: *90 calories*
2 slices whole wheat bread: *160 calories*
1 slice low-fat American cheese: *41 calories*
1 cup sliced apple: *64 calories*

Total: *355 calories*

Top bread with tuna and cheese and toast in a toaster oven. Enjoy apples on the side.

Snack (Women): 1 cup sliced pineapple: *78 calories*
Snack (Men): 1½ cups sliced pineapple and
1 piece of string cheese: *197 calories*

Dinner: Chicken Stir-Fry and Veggies

4 ounces boneless, skinless chicken breast: *192 calories*
1 large zucchini: *62 calories*
1 cup chopped carrots: *48 calories*
1 cup broccoli florets: *24 calories*
1 cup red peppers: *26 calories*
½ cup water: *0 calories*
Cooking spray: *7 calories*

Total: *359 calories*

Heat a wok or large skillet coated with cooking spray over medium-high heat. Add all ingredients and cook, stirring continuously until water has evaporated and ingredients are cooked.

Snack (Women): 100-calorie low-fat yogurt
Snack (Men): 100-calorie low-fat yogurt and
1 plain instant oatmeal packet: *200 calories*

PHASE IV: ADD THE FOLLOWING INGREDIENTS

Breakfast: 1 slice whole wheat toast = *80 additional calories*

Lunch: 1 slice low-fat American cheese (31 calories) and ½ cup apple (32 calories) = *63 additional calories*

Dinner: 1 ounce chicken breast (48 calories) and 1 cup broccoli florets (24 calories) = *72 additional calories*

(Women Total) Phase II: 1,295 calories / Phase IV: 1,510 calories
(Men Total) Phase II: 1,605 calories / Phase IV: 1,820 calories

PHASE II: DAY 18

Breakfast: Banana Graham

100-calorie low-fat banana yogurt
1 medium-size banana, sliced: *105 calories*
2 large graham cracker rectangles: *120 calories*

Total: *325 calories*

Crush graham crackers at the bottom of a bowl. Pour container of banana yogurt over the graham crackers. Top with banana slices.

Snack (Women): 1 piece of string cheese: *80 calories*
Snack (Men): 1 piece of string cheese and
1 medium-size apple: *167 calories*

Lunch: Chicken Saté

4 ounces boneless, skinless chicken breast: *192 calories*

¼ teaspoon curry powder: *2 calories*

1 tablespoon peanut butter: *95 calories*

¼ tablespoon soy sauce: *3 calories*

¼ teaspoon sugar: *4 calories*

Juice of half a lime: *10 calories*

1 cup cucumber: *14 calories*

4 large green lettuce leaves:. *6 calories*

10 grapes: *15 calories*

2 tablespoons hot water: *0 calories*

Total: *341 calories*

Place chicken on skewer and grill until opaque or cooked thoroughly. Whisk peanut butter, curry powder, soy sauce, sugar, and lime juice with very hot water until sauce is smooth. Wrap sliced chicken in lettuce leaves with sauce. Enjoy cucumber and grapes on the side.

Snack (Women): ¼ cup roasted peanuts: *107 calories*
Snack (Men): ½ cup roasted peanuts: *214 calories*

Dinner: Dijon Turkey Sandwich

2 slices whole wheat bread: *160 calories*

5 slices low-fat turkey: *57 calories*

½ cup chopped spinach: *4 calories*

1 cup sliced tomatoes: *38 calories*

2 teaspoons Dijon mustard: *10 calories*

1½ cups baby carrots: *60 calories*

Total: *329 calories*

Put all ingredients together between 2 slices of bread. Enjoy carrots on the side.

Snack (Women): ½ cup 2% cottage cheese: *90 calories*
Snack (Men): 1 cup 2% cottage cheese and
½ cup strawberries: *203 calories*

PHASE IV: ADD THE FOLLOWING INGREDIENTS

Breakfast: 1 large graham cracker rectangle = *60 additional calories*

Lunch: 1 ounce chicken breast (48 calories), ½ cup cucumber
(7 calories), and 10 grapes (15 calories) = *70 additional calories*

Dinner: 3 slices low-fat turkey (34 calories), ½ cup strawberries
(23 calories), and ½ cup baby carrots (20) = *77 additional calories*

(Women Total) Phase II: 1,272 calories / Phase IV: 1,479 calories
(Men Total) Phase II: 1,579 calories / Phase IV: 1,786 calories

PHASE II: DAY 19

Breakfast: Vegetable Omelet

4 egg whites: *60 calories*

1 cup chopped zucchini: *28 calories*

1 cup broccoli, cut into small florets: *24 calories*

1 cup chopped spinach: *8 calories*

1 ounce low-fat cheddar cheese: *90 calories*

1 orange: *65 calories*
1 cup sliced strawberries: *46 calories*
Cooking spray: *7 calories*

Total: *328 calories*

Combine egg whites, zucchini, and broccoli. Cook egg mixture over medium heat in a nonstick skillet coated with cooking spray. When the bottom side of the omelet is solid, flip or fold with a spatula and cook the other side.

Snack (Women): 1 celery stalk and
1 tablespoon peanut butter: *101 calories*
Snack (Men): 2 celery stalks and
2 tablespoons peanut butter: *202 calories*

Lunch: Shades of Green Tuna Salad

6 ounces canned tuna in water, drained: *180 calories*
2 tablespoons fat-free mayo: *44 calories*
1 cup chopped celery: *20 calories*
1 medium cucumber, seeded and diced: *39 calories*
1 cup chopped green pepper: *26 calories*
2 red-tipped lettuce leaves: *6 calories*

Total: *315 calories*

Stir together tuna, mayo, and veggies until combined. Serve over leaves of lettuce.

Snack (Women): 1 Laughing Cow Light Garlic & Herb cheese wedge and 3 Triscuits: *107 calories*
Snack (Men): 2 Laughing Cow Light Garlic & Herb cheese wedges and 3 Triscuits: *214 calories*

Dinner: Apricot Ginger Chicken

4 ounces boneless, skinless chicken breast: *192 calories*

1 teaspoon peeled, grated fresh ginger: *6 calories*

2 tablespoons apricot preserves: *96 calories*

¼ tablespoon cider vinegar: *1 calorie*

1 tablespoon chopped green onion: *4 calories*

1 teaspoon soy sauce: *3 calories*

1 cup green beans: *34 calories*

Total: *336 calories*

In small bowl, combine ginger, apricot preserves, vinegar, green onions, and soy sauce. Grill chicken, then brush with apricot sauce. Serve green beans separately.

Snack (Women): 100-calorie low-fat yogurt
Snack (Men): 100-calorie low-fat yogurt and 2 sliced kiwis:
192 calories

PHASE IV: ADD THE FOLLOWING INGREDIENTS

Breakfast: 2 egg whites (30 calories) and ½ ounce low-fat cheddar cheese (45 calories) = *75 additional calories*

Lunch: 2 ounces canned tuna (60 calories) and 2 red-tipped lettuce leaves (6 calories) = *66 additional calories*

Dinner: 1 ounce chicken breast (48 calories) and 1 cup green beans (34 calories) = *82 additional calories*

(Women Total) Phase II: 1,287 calories / Phase IV: 1,510 calories
(Men Total) Phase II: 1,587 calories / Phase IV: 1,810 calories

PHASE II: DAY 20

Breakfast: Spinach Scramble

1 cup chopped spinach: *8 calories*
2 egg whites: *30 calories*
1 tablespoon celery, minced: *1 calorie*
½ cup chopped tomatoes: *19 calories*
2 slices whole wheat bread: *160 calories*
1 ounce of feta cheese: *74 calories*
½ orange: *33 calories*
Cooking spray: *7 calories*
Pinch each of salt, pepper, nutmeg

Total: *332 calories*

Add spinach, celery, tomatoes, and feta to egg whites. Cook mixture over medium heat in nonstick skillet coated with cooking spray. Add salt, pepper, and nutmeg. Toast two slices of whole wheat bread and enjoy on the side with the orange half.

Snack (Women): 1 piece of string cheese: *80 calories*
Snack (Men): 2 pieces of string cheese: *160 calories*

Lunch: Rainbow Salad

3 cups spinach leaves: *24 calories*
1 cup mandarin orange sections: *33 calories*
1 cup sliced pineapple: *78 calories*
1 cup sliced strawberries: *46 calories*
1 cup diced apple: *64 calories*
10 almonds: *76 calories*

Total: *321 calories*

Mix all ingredients together in a large bowl.

Snack (Women): 1½ cups raspberries: *93 calories*
Snack (Men): 1½ cups raspberries and
1½ cups blueberries: *216 calories*

Dinner: Grilled Tuna with Tomato

6 ounces tuna steak: *246 calories*

1 cup cherry tomatoes: *38 calories*

1 tablespoon cilantro: *1 calorie*

1 tablespoon lemon juice: *5 calories*

1 cup fresh green beans: *34 calories*

12 asparagus spears: *48 calories*

Salt and pepper to taste

Total: *372 calories*

Cut tomatoes in half and combine with cilantro and lemon juice. Season with black pepper to taste. Grill tuna and top with tomato mixture. Serve green beans and asparagus on the side.

Snack (Women): 100-calorie low-fat yogurt
Snack (Men): 100-calorie low-fat yogurt and
1 plain instant oatmeal packet: *200 calories*

PHASE IV: ADD THE FOLLOWING INGREDIENTS

Breakfast: 2 egg whites (30 calories) and ½ ounce feta (37 calories) =
67 additional calories

Lunch: 10 almonds = *76 additional calories*

Dinner: 1 ounce tuna steak (41 calories) and 4 asparagus spears
(16 calories) = *57 additional calories*

(Women Total) Phase II: 1,298 calories / Phase IV: 1,498 calories
(Men Total) Phase II: 1,601 calories / Phase IV: 1,801 calories

PHASE II: DAY 21

Breakfast: MultiGrain Cheerios

1½ cups MultiGrain Cheerios: *168 calories*
1 cup 1% milk: *100 calories*
1½ cups sliced strawberries: *69 calories*

Total: *337 calories*

Serve Cheerios with milk and strawberries.

Snack (Women): ¼ cup of roasted peanuts: *107 calories*
Snack (Men): ½ cup of roasted peanuts: *214 calories*

Lunch: Grilled Pineapple Shrimp

6 ounces shrimp: *168 calories*
1 cup cubed pineapple: *78 calories*
¾ cup mango: *78 calories*

Total: *324 calories*

*Cut pineapple and mango into one-inch cubes and alternate on skewers
(if wood, soak in water for 30 minutes first) with shrimp, then grill.*

Snack (Women): 1 piece of string cheese: *80 calories*
Snack (Men): 1 piece of string cheese and
1 medium-size apple: *167 calories*

Dinner: Lemon Mushroom Herb Chicken

4 ounces boneless, skinless chicken breast: *192 calories*
1 cup sliced mushrooms: *18 calories*
¼ teaspoon basil: *0 calories*

¼ teaspoon oregano: *0 calories*

3 lemon slices: *6 calories*

½ cup wild rice: *83 calories*

1 cup green beans: *34 calories*

½ cup water: *0 calories*

Total: *333 calories*

In a small ovenproof dish, place chicken topped with mushrooms, lemon, and spices. Bake at 350 degrees for 30 minutes or until cooked through. While chicken is cooking, combine rice and water in saucepan, heat until boiling, then cook for 45 to 50 minutes over medium-low heat. Sprinkle basil and oregano over entire entrée. Steam green beans separately.

Snack (Women): ½ cup 2% cottage cheese and 1 medium tomato, sliced: *116 calories*
Snack (Men): 1 cup 2% cottage cheese and 1 medium tomato, sliced: *206 calories*

PHASE IV: ADD THE FOLLOWING INGREDIENTS

Breakfast: ½ cup Cheerios (56 calories) and ½ cup strawberries (23 calories) = *79 additional calories*

Lunch: 2 ounces shrimp = *56 additional calories*

Dinner: 1 ounce chicken breast (48 calories) and ½ cup green beans (17 calories) = *65 additional calories*

(Women Total) Phase II: 1,297 calories / Phase IV: 1,497 calories
(Men Total) Phase II: 1,581 calories / Phase IV: 1,781 calories

PHASE II: DAY 22

Breakfast: Pineapple Toast

1 cup 2% cottage cheese: *180 calories*
1 cup pineapple: *78 calories*
1 slice whole wheat toast: *80 calories*

Total: *338 calories*

Mix diced pineapple and cottage cheese. Serve on top of toast or separately.

Snack (Women): 2 large kiwis, sliced: *110 calories*
Snack (Men): 2 large kiwis, sliced, and
½ cup 2% cottage cheese: *310 calories*

Lunch: Tortilla Roll-Up

3 pieces low-fat turkey bacon, chopped: *69 calories*
½ cup chopped green pepper: *26 calories*
⅛ teaspoon ground cumin: *3 calories*
2 egg whites: *30 calories*
½ cup chopped tomato: *19 calories*
1 ounce low-fat cheddar cheese: *90 calories*
Fat-free flour tortilla: *100 calories*

Total: *337 calories*

In a medium nonstick skillet, cook bacon until crisp. Add green pepper and cumin. Cook for 3 minutes. Add egg whites and cook for 2 minutes. Stir in tomato. Spoon onto tortilla, sprinkle with cheese, and roll up.

Snack (Women): 1 hard-boiled egg: *90 calories*
Snack (Men): 2 hard-boiled eggs: *180 calories*

Dinner: Lemon Chicken

5 ounces boneless, skinless chicken breast: *240 calories*
4 lemon slices: *8 calories*
1 cup green beans: *34 calories*
1 large zucchini: *62 calories*
Pinch each of dried basil and oregano

Total: *344 calories*

In a small ovenproof dish, place chicken topped with lemon and spices. Bake chicken at 350 degrees for 30 minutes or until cooked through. Steam sliced zucchini and green beans separately.

Snack (Women): 1 Laughing Cow Light Garlic & Herb cheese wedge and 3 Triscuits: *107 calories*
Snack (Men): 2 Laughing Cow Light Garlic & Herb cheese wedges and 6 Triscuits: *214 calories*

PHASE IV: ADD THE FOLLOWING INGREDIENTS

Breakfast: 1 slice whole wheat toast = *80 additional calories*

Lunch: 4 pieces low-fat turkey (23 calories), 2 egg whites from hard-boiled egg (30 calories), and ¼ cup green peppers (13 calories) = *66 additional calories*

Dinner: 1 ounce chicken breast (48 calories) and ½ cup green beans (17 calories) = *65 additional calories*

(Women Total) Phase II: 1,326 calories / Phase IV: 1,537 calories
(Men Total) Phase II: 1,723 calories / Phase IV: 1,934 calories

PHASE II: DAY 23

Breakfast: Hot Oatmeal with Fruit

1 packet microwavable oatmeal: *103 calories*

1 medium pear, diced: *98 calories*

1½ cups diced apple: *98 calories*

Total: *299 calories*

Add water and microwave oatmeal for time indicated. Mix together apple and pear for fruit salad.

Snack (Women): ½ cup 2% cottage cheese: *90 calories*

Snack (Men): 1 cup 2% cottage cheese: *180 calories*

Lunch: Chicken Greek Salad

4 ounces boneless, skinless chicken breast: *192 calories*

½ cup chopped tomato: *19 calories*

½ cup seeded, diced cucumber: *7 calories*

¾ teaspoon lemon juice: *3 calories*

½ teaspoon oregano: *0 calories*

1 ounce feta cheese: *74 calories*

4 large black olives, halved: *16 calories*

3 cups mixed greens: *24 calories*

Total: *335 calories*

Combine all ingredients in bowl and serve.

Snack (Women): 1 large celery stalk and
1 tablespoon peanut butter: *101 calories*

Snack (Men): 2 large celery stalks and
2 tablespoons peanut butter: *202 calories*

Dinner: Stir-Fried Shrimp and Veggies

6 ounces precooked shrimp: *168 calories*
1 large zucchini: *62 calories*
1 cup sliced carrots: *48 calories*
1 cup broccoli florets: *24 calories*
1 cup sliced green or red peppers: *26 calories*
Cooking spray: *7 calories*
½ cup water: *0 calories*

Total: *335 calories*

Heat wok or large skillet coated with cooking spray over medium-high heat. Add water, shrimp, and vegetables and cook, stirring continuously until water has evaporated and ingredients are cooked.

Snack (Women): 1 piece of string cheese: *80 calories*
Snack (Men): 1 piece of string cheese and
⅓ cup raisins: *208 calories*

PHASE IV: ADD THE FOLLOWING INGREDIENTS

Breakfast: 1 cup sliced apple = *65 additional calories*

Lunch: 1 ounce chicken breast (48 calories) and ½ ounce feta (37 calories) = *85 additional calories*

Dinner: 2 ounces cooked shrimp (56 calories) and 1 cup sliced red or green pepper (26 calories) = *82 additional calories*

(Women Total) Phase II: 1,240 calories / Phase IV: 1,472 calories
(Men Total) Phase II: 1,559 calories / Phase IV: 1,791 calories

PHASE II: DAY 24

Breakfast: Raisin Bran Cereal

1 cup raisin bran: *186 calories*
1 cup 1% milk: *100 calories*
1 cup strawberries: *48 calories*

Total: *334 calories*

Serve cereal with milk and fruit.

Snack (Women): ½ cup 2% cottage cheese and
2 peach slices: *109 calories*
Snack (Men): 1 cup 2% cottage cheese and
2 peach slices: *199 calories*

Lunch: Chicken Sandwich

2 slices whole wheat toast: *160 calories*
4 slices low-fat chicken: *46 calories*
2 tomato slices: *8 calories*
2 romaine lettuce leaves: *3 calories*
1 slice low-fat American cheese: *31 calories*
1 cup blueberries: *82 calories*

Total: *330 calories*

Combine all ingredients between 2 slices of wheat toast. Enjoy blueberries on the side.

Snack (Women): 1 large celery stalk and
1 tablespoon peanut butter: *101 calories*
Snack (Men): 2 large celery stalks and
2 tablespoons peanut butter: *202 calories*

Dinner: Poached Salmon and Broccoli

6 ounces skinless poached salmon fillet: *240 calories*

1 cup broccoli florets: *24 calories*

1 cup chopped carrots: *48 calories*

¼ cup water: *0 calories*

¼ teaspoon salt

Total: *312 calories*

Place salmon in eight-by-eight-inch glass baking dish. Sprinkle with salt. Add water to dish. Cover and cook in microwave on high 8 minutes or until fish just turns opaque throughout and flakes easily when tested with a fork.

Snack (Women): 12 almonds: *91 calories*
Snack (Men): 25 almonds: *190 calories*

PHASE IV: ADD THE FOLLOWING INGREDIENTS

Breakfast: 1 slice of whole wheat toast = *80 additional calories*

Lunch: 1 cup blueberries = *82 additional calories*

Dinner: 1 ounce salmon (40 calories) and
1 cup broccoli florets (24 calories) = *64 additional calories*

(Women Total) Phase II: 1,277 calories / Phase IV: 1,503 calories
(Men Total) Phase II: 1,567 calories / Phase IV: 1,793 calories

PHASE II: DAY 25

Breakfast: Cottage Cheese and Fruit

1 cup sliced apple: *64 calories*

½ cup blueberries: *41 calories*

1 cup strawberries: *46 calories*
1 cup 2% cottage cheese: *180 calories*

Total: *331 calories*

Combine all ingredients in a bowl and serve.

Snack (Women): 10 cashew nuts: *91 calories*
Snack (Men): 20 cashew nuts: *182 calories*

Lunch: Fagioli Soup and Salad

1 cup canned diced tomatoes: *50 calories*
1 cup cooked canned kidney beans: *190 calories*
¼ cup chopped carrots: *12 calories*
1 cup fresh green beans: *34 calories*
2 cups mixed greens: *16 calories*
½ cup sliced cucumber: *7 calories*
1 tablespoon balsamic vinegar: *10 calories*
1½ cups water: *0 calories*

Total: *319 calories*

Combine water, tomatoes, kidney beans, carrots, and green beans in medium-size saucepan. Simmer for 10 minutes. For salad, combine greens and cucumber and drizzle with balsamic vinegar.

Snack (Women): 100-calorie low-fat yogurt and
½ cup strawberries: *124 calories*
Snack (Men): 100-calorie low-fat yogurt,
1 cup strawberries, and 1 cup blueberries: *228 calories*

Dinner: Grilled Chicken and Veggies

4 ounces boneless, skinless chicken breast: *192 calories*
1 large zucchini, chopped: *62 calories*

1 cup broccoli florets: *24 calories*

1 medium yellow squash: *27 calories*

½ teaspoon dried basil and

½ teaspoon dried oregano (combined): *5 calories*

Total: *310 calories*

Grill chicken until cooked through. Steam vegetables and top with basil and oregano.

Snack (Women): 1 piece of string cheese: *80 calories*
Snack (Men): 1 piece of string cheese and
1 medium-size apple: *167 calories*

PHASE IV: ADD THE FOLLOWING INGREDIENTS

Breakfast: ½ cup 2% cottage cheese = *90 additional calories*

Lunch: ¼ cup kidney beans (48 calories), ¼ cup carrots (12 calories), and ½ cup green beans (17 calories) = *77 additional calories*

Dinner: 1 ounce chicken breast (48 calories) and 1 cup broccoli florets (24 calories) = *72 additional calories*

(Women Total) Phase II: 1,255 calories / Phase IV: 1,494 calories
(Men Total) Phase II: 1,537 calories / Phase IV: 1,776 calories

PHASE II: DAY 26

Breakfast: Eggs and Blueberries

2 eggs: *180 calories*

1 cup blueberries: *82 calories*

1 cup sliced apple: *64 calories*

Total: *326 calories*

Hard-boil 2 eggs. Serve with fruit.

Snack (Women): 100-calorie low-fat yogurt
Snack (Men): 100-calorie low-fat yogurt and
2 medium kiwis, sliced: *192 calories*

Lunch: Baked Potato Topped with Salsa and Cottage Cheese

1 medium potato: *220 calories*
¼ cup salsa: *10 calories*
½ cup 2% cottage cheese: *90 calories*

Total: *320 calories*

Preheat oven to 350 degrees. Take one potato and poke holes in it with a fork about ten times. Place potato directly on oven rack and cook for 1 hour and 15 minutes. Top with cottage cheese and salsa.

Snack (Women): 1 piece of string cheese: *80 calories*
Snack (Men): 2 pieces of string cheese: *160 calories*

Dinner: Chicken Fajita

4 ounces boneless, skinless chicken breast: *192 calories*
1 cup chopped green pepper: *26 calories*
4 tablespoons tomato juice: *10 calories*
1 teaspoon chili powder: *8 calories*
1 teaspoon garlic powder: *12 calories*
2 corn tortillas: *90 calories*
Cooking spray: *7 calories*

Total: *345 calories*

In large nonstick skillet coated with cooking spray, combine chicken, peppers, tomato juice, chili powder, and garlic powder; cook over medium-high heat until chicken is cooked through; put chicken mixture into tortillas and serve.

Snack (Women): 2 Reduced-Fat Wheat Thins crackers and 1 tablespoon peanut butter: *120 calories*
Snack (Men): 4 Reduced-Fat Wheat Thins crackers and 2 tablespoons peanut butter: *240 calories*

PHASE IV: ADD THE FOLLOWING INGREDIENTS

Breakfast: 1 hard-boiled egg = *90 additional calories*

Lunch: 1 cup carrots = *48 additional calories*

Dinner: 1 ounce chicken breast (48 calories) and 1 cup sliced green pepper (26 calories) = *74 additional calories*

(Women Total) Phase II: 1,291 calories / Phase IV: 1,503 calories
(Men Total) Phase II: 1,583 calories / Phase IV: 1,795 calories

PHASE II: DAY 27

Breakfast: Turkey Sandwich

2 pieces whole wheat bread: *160 calories*

4 slices low-fat turkey: *46 calories*

1 slice tomato: *8 calories*

1 leaf romaine lettuce: *2 calories*

1 slice low-fat American cheese: *41 calories*

1 cup blueberries: *82 calories*

Total: *339 calories*

Place turkey, tomato, lettuce, and cheese between 2 slices of bread. Enjoy blueberries on the side.

Snack (Women): 12 cashews: *109 calories*
Snack (Men): 25 cashews: *228 calories*

Lunch: Mozzarella Veggies

1 cup diced carrots: *48 calories*

2 cups broccoli florets: *48 calories*

1 cup diced zucchini: *28 calories*

1 cup diced yellow squash: *28 calories*

1 cup diced green pepper: *26 calories*

1 cup bean sprouts: *30 calories*

¼ cup chickpeas: *67 calories*

1 ounce low-fat mozzarella cheese: *72 calories*

2 quarts water: *0 calories*

Total: *347 calories*

Fill four-quart saucepan half full of water and boil. Add veggies to boiling water and cook until tender. Place vegetables on a plate or in a bowl. Sprinkle mozzarella cheese and chickpeas over vegetables.

Snack (Women): 1 nectarine: *67 calories*
Snack (Men): 1 nectarine and
1 packet of plain instant oatmeal: *167 calories*

Dinner: Ginger Flounder Fillet

7 ounces flounder fillet: *182 calories*

2 teaspoons ginger: *12 calories*

2 tablespoons fresh basil, sliced: *22 calories*

2 cups broccoli florets: *48 calories*

1 large zucchini: *62 calories*

Cooking spray: *7 calories*

Total: *333 calories*

Coat nonstick twelve-inch skillet with cooking spray and heat over medium-high until hot. Add fish and ginger to skillet and cook until flounder is opaque and flakes easily with a fork, about 5 minutes per side. Add basil at end. Steam broccoli and zucchini.

Snack (Women): ½ cup 2% cottage cheese: *90 calories*
Snack (Men): 1 cup 2% cottage cheese: *180 calories*

PHASE IV: ADD THE FOLLOWING INGREDIENTS

Breakfast: 1 cup blueberries = *82 additional calories*

Lunch: 1 cup squash (28 calories) and
1 cup zucchini (28 calories) = *56 additional calories*

Dinner: 2 ounces flounder fillet = *52 additional calories*

(Women Total) Phase II: 1,285 calories / Phase IV: 1,475 calories
(Male Total) Phase II: 1,594 calories / Phase IV: 1,784 calories

PHASE II: DAY 28

Breakfast: Special K Cereal with Milk

1 cup Special K cereal: *115 calories*
1 cup 1% milk: *100 calories*
½ cup strawberries: *23 calories*
100-calorie low-fat yogurt

Total: *338 calories*

Pour cereal into bowl and cover with milk.

Snack (Women): 1 piece of string cheese: *80 calories*
Snack (Men): 1 piece of string cheese and 20 almonds: *232 calories*

Lunch: Vegetables and Brown Rice

1 cup brown rice: *220 calories*

1 cup chopped celery: *20 calories*

1 cup sliced mushrooms: *18 calories*

1 cup chopped carrots: *48 calories*

1 cup broccoli florets: *24 calories*

2 tablespoons soy sauce: *20 calories*

2 tablespoons water: *0 calories*

Total: *350 calories*

Steam or stir-fry vegetables with soy sauce and water. Serve over rice.

Snack (Women): 4 slices Sara Lee honey ham with
2 teaspoons honey mustard, rolled in lettuce leaf: *72 calories*
Snack (Men): 8 slices Sara Lee honey ham with
4 teaspoons honey mustard, rolled in lettuce leaf: *145 calories*

Dinner: Halibut and Broccoli

4 ounces halibut: *124 calories*

2 cups broccoli florets: *48 calories*

1 cup spinach leaves: *8 calories*

½ cup 2% cottage cheese: *90 calories*

1 nectarine, sliced: *67 calories*

Total: *337 calories*

Grill halibut until cooked. Steam broccoli and spinach and serve with fish. Mix cottage cheese with nectarine and serve on side.

Snack (Women): 1 large celery stalk and
1 tablespoon peanut butter: *101 calories*
Snack (Men): 2 large celery stalks and
2 tablespoons peanut butter: *202 calories*

PHASE IV: ADD THE FOLLOWING INGREDIENTS

Breakfast: ½ cup Special K = *57 additional calories*

Lunch: 1 cup carrots (48 calories), 1 cup broccoli (24 calories), and 1 tablespoon soy sauce (10 calories) = *82 additional calories*

Dinner: 2 ounces halibut (62 calories) and 1 cup spinach (8 calories) = *70 additional calories*

(Women Total) Phase II: 1,278 calories / Phase IV: 1,487 calories
(Men Total) Phase II: 1,604 calories / Phase IV: 1,813 calories

CHAPTER 12

Eating Out While
Cardio-Free

We are all eating out, taking out, and ordering in more than ever before. According to the U.S. Department of Agriculture, we are eating one-third of all meals out, up from 18 percent in the 1970s. Eating out and ordering in are just a function of our busy, modern-day lives, and convenience has become key. Not surprisingly, Tufts University research shows that those who eat out are more likely to have more body fat. Marion Nestle, a New York University professor of nutrition, states that "the big problem will still be calories and that portion sizes are so large."

When it comes to calories, anything that you do not prepare yourself is suspect. Mom, who has the best of intentions, probably doesn't realize that her green bean casserole has thousands of calories or her beautiful, healthy-looking salad is topped with 900 calories of cheese, croutons, bacon bits, and dressing. Even dietitians, who determine calorie counts for a living, underestimated restaurant calories 37 percent and fat by 49 percent in studies conducted by New York University. The reason is that prepared food, especially restaurant food, is packed with hidden fats, calories, and sodium. You can eat just about anywhere and stay on your plan, but only if you navigate the menu with a very clear strategy.

Here are the best strategies to keep the calories down while eating out.

BREAKFAST

Do order:

• two poached eggs (90 calories per egg) and a slice of whole wheat toast (80 calories per slice) with a little jam (18 calories per teaspoon): 300 calories. NOTE: Even egg white omelets (15 calories per egg white) are frequently made with lots of butter (100 calories per tablespoon) or other added fat. Very few places make the omelet with a nonstick cooking spray, which is what I do at home. For this reason, I'd skip it.

• whole grain cereal (for example, 110 calories per cup of Cheerios) with 1 percent milk (100 calories per cup) and one cup of strawberries (46 calories per cup): approximately 300 calories

• oatmeal (plain instant oatmeal packets are about 100 calories)

• fresh fruit (62 calories per cup of raspberries or 82 calories per cup of blueberries) and 2 percent cottage cheese (180 calories per cup): approximately 300 calories

Be careful when ordering:

• pancakes, waffles, Danishes (340 calories for a Dunkin' Donuts cheese Danish), muffins (which are cake in disguise and will run you 470 calories for a blueberry muffin at Dunkin' Donuts), and doughnuts (*fried cake*, which will run to more than 200 calories at Dunkin' Donuts).

• croissants (which are filled with butter), which could be between 300 and 500 calories each, especially the big ones.

• big bagels with real cream cheese (100 calories per ounce). A 200-calorie bagel is fine, but when eating out, they are generally huge, more like 500 calories, and that is before the cream cheese.

LUNCH

Do order:

• a low-fat turkey (11 calories per slice) sandwich on whole wheat bread (80 calories per slice) with lettuce (1 calorie per slice), tomato (3 calories per thin slice), and mustard. Always ask for mustard, which is 5 calories per tablespoon, never mayo (100 calories per tablespoon, unless it is low calorie): approximately 320 calories

• a salad (8 calories per cup of mixed greens, but never a Caesar; see below in the Dinner section) with grilled chicken (48 calories per ounce) or shrimp (28 calories per ounce) and low-calorie dressing (24 calories per tablespoon for low-cal ranch) or balsamic vinegar (10 calories per tablespoon) on the side (dressing should *always* be on the side): approximately 300 calories

• poached eggs (90 calories per egg) and whole wheat toast (80 calories per slice) and jam (18 calories per teaspoon of jam): approximately 300 calories

Be careful when ordering:

• soup: Most restaurant soup is loaded with calories, fat, and sodium. Many people assume that soup is low in calories, but they are terribly wrong. If you must have some, please limit the portion to a cup instead of a bowl. (For example, Corner Bakery's Loaded Baked Potato soup is 650 calories per serving, and the Cheddar Broccoli soup is 460 calories per serving.)

• mayonnaise-based salads, such as tuna, chicken, or egg salads. They can easily be 700 to 800 calories per serving (for example, if you order a tuna salad sandwich from Panera Bread it runs 720 calories!). NOTE: In the New York University dietitian study cited earlier, the average estimate for a tuna fish sandwich was 375 calories, when in reality it was 720 calories—almost double!

• chili, which is generally very high in calories because a restaurant doesn't drain off all the fat from the meat as you would do (I hope) at home. This is why it generally tastes so good. A 7.5-ounce can of store-bought chili, however, is about 300 to 325 calories and is perfectly acceptable.

DINNER

For dinner, the strategies are broken down by the types of restaurants most frequented by American diners. I have heard some experts recommend that you order appetizers for entrées, but let's be honest, nobody does that with any regularity. Furthermore, some appetizers are even higher in calories than entrées. So I advise you to be very clear when ordering and ask the waiter lots of questions if there is something that you don't understand. The more informed you are, the better your chances of "calorically" surviving eating out.

Steak Houses

People are always shocked when I tell them that you can get some of the best low-calorie, high-flavor foods at a steak house. Sure, there are twenty-seven-ounce porterhouse steaks (which run between 60 and 90 calories per ounce) and baked potatoes (220 calories for a medium-size one) brimming with sour cream (26 calories per tablespoon), cheese (110 calories per ounce of cheddar), and bacon bits (30 calories per tablespoon), but these restaurants also carry great seafood, the highest quality produce, and many options that are both low in calories and satisfying.

Appetizers

Always order a shrimp cocktail (28 calories per ounce of shrimp and 15 calories per tablespoon of cocktail sauce). It is low in calories, very tasty, and a great source of protein.

Or order a chopped salad (8 calories per cup of mixed greens) with half the cheese (use low-fat if possible, which is still 90 calories per ounce) or no cheese, and dressing on the side (again, balsamic vinegar is 10 calories per tablespoon, or low-fat ranch dressing is 24 calories per tablespoon).

Be careful with Caesar salad (Wishbone Caesar dressing is 85 calories per tablespoon, and croutons run about 70 calories per half ounce). I always say, "Brutus killed Caesar, but Caesar is killing you!" Most estimates of this salad are around 750 calories, and it is the most frequently ordered salad in the country.

Entrées

Order any of the fish options grilled (40 calories per ounce of salmon and 41 calories per ounce of tuna, for example) with very little olive oil (120 calories per tablespoon) or, ideally, poached. Fish is generally 30–45 calories an ounce, so make sure to inquire about the size.

Or order a small filet of about eight ounces (lean beef is around 60 calories an ounce, so you may have to share or ask the waiter to wrap up half the order, which would be great the next day sliced over a salad). Please make sure that the filet does not have butter (100 calories per tablespoon) on top, and trim off all the visible fat.

Sides

Order any of the fresh vegetables steamed—not sautéed, creamed, or anything with added fat (24 calories per cup of broccoli, 46 calories per cup of carrots, and 4 calories per asparagus spear).

Go for the plain baked potato (220 calories) and just sprinkle on some salt and pepper (5 calories per teaspoon) for additional flavor. For the record, baked potatoes do have a high glycemic index, but when the other choices are fries (570 calories for large fries at McDonald's), twice-baked potatoes (easily double the calories of a plain baked), and other buttered, fat-drenched potatoes, the plain baked potato comes out as the obvious winner. Plus, when you couple it with the fish (30–40 calories per ounce) or beef (60 calories per ounce of lean beef), the glycemic index of the potato is offset.

MEXICAN RESTAURANTS

Some research indicates that spice can increase your metabolism slightly, and while eating out, every little bit helps. That's why you sometimes sweat when you eat something spicy.

Appetizers

Skip the chips (320 calories for a handful, which are always fried), and order some flour tortillas (about 60 calories each) to eat with the salsa (6 calories per tablespoon).

Order a salad (8 calories per cup) with dressing on the side (10 calories per tablespoon of balsamic vinegar, or 24 calories per tablespoon of low-fat dressing), use the salsa instead of the dressing, or squeeze lots of lime (10 calories for half a lime) on top. Adding squeezed lime to anything is a tasty option.

Entrées

Your absolute best bet is to order shrimp (28 calories per ounce), chicken (48 calories per ounce), or beef (60 calories per ounce) fajitas, and specifically ask for them to be cooked in very little oil (120 calories per tablespoon). They will come with flour tortillas (60 calories each), but if you've already had a few with your salsa, it is best to skip them.

Careful when ordering the burrito, which is filled with cheese (100 calories per ounce of cheddar), refried beans (100 calories per quarter cup), guacamole (see below), and probably lots of other high-fat foods that you are not aware of. At El Pollo Loco in Irvine, California, the Ultimate Chicken Burrito is 702 calories. And a loaded taco salad could be as high as 1,100 calories. You would think that would be a lower-calorie choice, but the refried beans, guacamole, sour cream (26 calories per tablespoon), *and* the shell add up to almost a whole day's worth of calories.

Your Diet Busters

The refried beans in restaurants are often made with lard (but the ones you purchase at the store are only around 120 calories for 4 ounces, but a little high in sodium, as are all canned products). The rice (110 calories per half cup of plain brown rice, and 80 calories per half cup of plain white rice) is made with butter or other fats that you would skip (I hope) if you prepared it at home.

Guacamole. Did you know that it can be close to 100 calories for a single chip with guacamole on top? Guacamole should be eaten the way you would eat butter (100 calories per tablespoon): A little bit should go a very long way.

ITALIAN RESTAURANTS

It is tough to get the calories out of a lot of Italian foods because of one simple ingredient: olive oil. Yes, it is healthier in terms of good fat than the other oils, but it still has 120 calories a tablespoon, as all oils do.

Appetizers

Order grilled calamari (26 calories per ounce), light on the olive oil.
Or order a salad (8 calories per cup of mixed greens) with dressing

(balsamic vinegar is 10 calories per tablespoon, and low-fat dressings run around 24 calories per tablespoon) on the side. Another good option is polenta (106 calories per half cup). It's cornmeal; it's tasty, and low in calories.

To be safe, be careful when ordering the antipasto platter, as it is generally swimming in oil.

Entrées

Order fish (30–45 calories per ounce) grilled in very little olive oil.

Your best bet is to avoid eating pasta (or eat it less often), but if you just can't do this, proceed with caution. The problem is not so much the noodles, but the fact that virtually all restaurants toss them in oil or butter (the latter is 100 calories per tablespoon) before they put on the sauce. Also, the portions are often huge. Two ounces of cooked pasta is around 150 calories. Most restaurant portions are at least four times that size. For the record, estimates of fettuccine Alfredo come in as high as 1,500 calories. Ouch!

Sides

Order steamed spinach (8 calories per cup), asparagus (4 calories per spear), or any other vegetable (24 calories per cup of broccoli).

NOTE: Pizza is loaded with calories and fat. One-quarter of a Tombstone frozen cheese pizza is 330 calories. Two slices of a medium hand-tossed cheese pizza at Pizza Hut is 518 calories. However, you can order pizza with one-half the cheese (even Domino's will do that) and always select vegetable toppings (for example: 13 calories for a half cup peppers, 4 calories for half a cup of spinach, 19 calories for a half cup tomato). Always blot the pizza with your napkin before eating it—you won't believe the amount of fat you will remove. If you order a salad (8 calories per cup of mixed greens) with dressing (10 calories per tablespoon for balsamic vinegar, and 24 calories for low-fat dressing) on the side to start, you won't be so quick to dive into the pizza ravenously!

CHINESE AND THAI RESTAURANTS

The key is to manage the sauce.

Appetizers

Order the soft steamed spring rolls (25 calories or so for each roll). They are very tasty and low in calories, but be careful with the plum sauce (45 calories per ounce).

Do order the chicken satay (48 calories an ounce) at a Thai restaurant, but severely limit the peanut sauce (150 calories per quarter cup).

Best to stay away from the fried egg rolls (150–200 calories per egg roll) or, at the very least, cut them in half.

Entrées

The first thing you must order is steamed vegetables (examples: 1 cup carrots is 46 calories; 1 cup broccoli is 24 calories) with chicken (48 calories per ounce), shrimp (26 calories per ounce), or beef (60 calories per ounce).

Order beef (60 calories per ounce) and broccoli (24 calories per cup), as it is generally made with a light garlic sauce (approximately 18 calories per tablespoon).

Be careful ordering the kung pao chicken. According to an article in the *Wall Street Journal*, it typically has 1,620 calories, which is more than most people should be eating all day.

Careful when ordering the pad thai. It tastes so good because the noodles are coated in sugar (46 calories per tablespoon) and peanut oil (120 calories per tablespoon), it's fried, and it has lots of peanuts (160 calories per ounce) on top. Peanuts are calorically dense, and while they are healthy for the body (if you recall, I have them in my eating plan), a little goes a long way. With all of these ingredients, pad thai can total 1,000 calories or more.

TIP: If you just love to order in stir-fried Chinese chicken with veggies and it does come in a brown sauce, here is what I want you to do:

1. Order two entrées, one steamed and the other in the brown sauce.

2. Fill your plate with half of the order of steamed veggies and chicken.

3. Place all the stir-fried Chinese chicken with veggies in a strainer (if you are in the restaurant, pick off most of the chicken and veggies from the top) and let most of the sauce drain through.

4. Place half of the stir-fried order on top of the steamed order and mix it all together. That way, you get the taste you like without all the added calories.

Sides

Brown rice (110 calories per half cup) is the better option, except I find it is frequently made with butter in the restaurant to add moisture. Ask your waiter if you can have it steamed—if not, then go with the white rice (80 calories per half cup). Similar to the baked potato, eating the white rice with protein will bring down its glycemic index.

GREEK RESTAURANTS

As I spent the majority of my childhood eating at Greek restaurants, I have a lot of knowledge regarding this food. My father was an accountant, so we always went to his clients' restaurants for dinner, and since we are Greek, most of his clients were as well. As with Italian food, you are once again playing "dodge the olive oil" (120 calories per tablespoon), as it is on virtually everything.

Appetizers

Do order the Greek salad with dressing on the side (8 calories per cup of mixed greens, 8 calories per tablespoon of balsamic vinegar). Feta cheese is 74 calories an ounce.

THE CARDIO-FREE DIET

Do order the grilled calamari (26 calories per ounce) with light oil (120 calories per tablespoon).

Careful when ordering anything with phyllo dough (85 calories per ounce), such as spinach pie or cheese triangles. I watched my grand-mother make these for years and they are loaded with butter—that's why they taste so good! Also, be very leery of the stuffed grape leaves. Many recipes can run from 300 to 700 calories per serving, but these numbers can differ dramatically in restaurants. They are generally made with a great deal of oil, both on the inside and out.

Entrées

Do order the grilled, boneless breast of chicken kebob (48 calories per ounce) with vegetables (46 calories per cup of carrots, 24 calories per cup of broccoli). Or order fish (30–45 calories per ounce) grilled with a little olive oil—it's excellent!

Careful when ordering anything with an unknown sauce, as it is gen-erally a combination of egg (90 calories per egg), lemon (9 calories per half a lemon), butter, and oil.

Sides

Okay to order: the big boiled potatoes that have a little bit of olive oil on top. Again, the protein and vegetables bring down the glycemic index of the potato.

Steamed spinach (8 calories per cup) is a good choice—all Greek restau-rants have spinach, even if it's not on the menu. Careful with the rice (80 calories per half cup) as it is filled with oil and butter and is very shiny.

Finally, restaurants want their food to taste good, and fat adds flavor. Even the healthier options are likely to be hiding butter, oil, cream (44 calories per tablespoon), and salt. The trick is to navigate both the menu and the waiter. Think of the waiter as your ambassador to leaner living, and tell him you appreciate his extra efforts and those of the chef to limit the fat and calories in your food. When you receive your food exactly as you ordered it, tip graciously. Nothing guarantees that a waiter will be on your side more than a fat tip, which is so much better than a fat you.

FAST FOOD

Almost every major chain now lists the calorie counts of each and every item on their website. If you are frequenting fast food restaurants, there is a way to stay on plan and not get in trouble. A few years back I wrote an article for *Good Housekeeping* magazine called "The Fast Food Diet." In it I described healthy options for breakfast, lunch, and dinner. Many readers e-mailed, faxed, and wrote to me saying, "How can you recommend fast food? It's so unhealthy!" Well, that is true and that is false.

It is a fact that we are all winding up at fast food restaurants from time to time, whether by choice or by necessity. Therefore, why not have a strategy to deal with that inevitability? Some of the food is pretty awful, and honestly, some is not so bad. Here are some of my recommendations, but I do still urge you to go directly to the site and print all the calorie counts. That way, you can make educated ordering decisions. Keep the pages in the glove compartment of your car—odds are, you will be driving there.

Breakfast

• **McDonald's:** The Egg McMuffin (300 calories), or the plain English muffin (I doubt it's whole wheat) and two scrambled eggs (360 calories).

• **Burger King:** Croissan'wich with egg and cheese (350 calories and yes, the croissant is probably filled with butter, but the calorie count is just a little high).

• **Subway:** All breakfast sandwiches on the healthy side are between 300 and 350 calories.

Lunch and Dinner

- **McDonald's:** Chicken McNuggets are 41 calories each (so you can have six or seven); a small burger is 290 calories.

- **Subway:** Seven of their six-inch sandwiches are 230–320 calories each.

- **Wendy's:** Ultimate Chicken Grill sandwich is 370 calories.

- **Taco Bell:** The plain bean burrito is 370 calories.

I know the last two are a little high, but they're the best options for those restaurants. The more you get into the habit of ordering lower-calorie options when eating fast food, the more you will succeed with this eating plan.

CHAPTER 13

The Seven Rules for Living Cardio-Free

I want to make sure you do everything you can to optimize your results, so here are a few additional suggestions to complement The Cardio-Free Diet.

YOU SNOOZE, YOU LOSE

The average American is sleeping two hours less than he or she did forty years ago. This is a big problem if you are trying to lose weight. Sleep causes two very important hormones to be produced. The first one, leptin, is a hormone that tells the body, "I'm getting full," which, as discussed in Chapter 10, is also produced when you eat foods that contain fat. The second hormone is ghrelin, sometimes called the hunger hormone. It tells the body, "Feed me." University of Chicago researchers restricted a group of men to only four hours of sleep a night. After as few as two nights, the men showed an 18 percent decrease in the amount of leptin and a 28 percent increase in ghrelin. Another case study showed that those who sleep fewer than seven hours were more likely to be obese than those who slept for seven or more. Insufficient sleep has also been linked to an increase in the stress hormone cortisol, which is catabolic (muscle-depleting), and can cause bingeing and increased hunger. And one more point: We all know what we do when we stay up late. We eat! Go to bed, and you may find the pounds coming off much faster.

WATER UP, WEIGHT DOWN

I know you have heard this before, but it's good advice. Research has shown that body fat is more efficiently burned for fuel in a well-hydrated environment. It's misleading to recommend the typical "eight, eight-ounce glasses a day," because your water needs are affected by the following factors:

- **Your weight:** More weight requires more water.

- **Your activity level:** More activity requires more water.

- **Your climate:** You require more water in a dry climate, but you also need more water in cold winters, when you are inside more with blasting dry heat. Buying a humidifier is a great decision during those cold months, and you will feel so much better in the morning when you have slept in a more humid environment.

- **Your sodium intake:** Sodium robs your body of water, so increase your water intake if you know you are consuming more sodium or simply eating out more (most chefs have a heavy hand with the salt). Also note that most restaurant soups are loaded with sodium.

- **Your alcohol consumption:** Alcohol dehydrates the body when it is broken down. As I urged you in Chapter 10, be a two-fisted drinker and consume two ounces of water for every ounce of alcohol. You will drink less and thank me in the morning!

- **Medication:** Certain medications are dehydrating, such as a diuretic for high blood pressure.

- **Cabin pressure:** Flying is very dehydrating, and you should drink as much water as possible when in the air. Some reports say that you can lose thirty-two ounces an hour while in an airplane.

I say to my clients that they should keep drinking water all day. If you are feeling thirsty, then you are already down about thirty-two ounces, so don't wait until you feel thirsty. People commonly say to me, "I just can't drink water. I am bloated enough as it is." News flash: You are bloated because you are terribly dehydrated. Since you are not giving your body water, the very smart brain tells it to hold on to the reserves in the outer tissues of your body. Therefore, you look and feel bloated. The moment you start drinking water, your brain will say, "We found water—release the reserves!" If you wear a ring, do the ring test. If the ring is tight, you are dehydrated. Drink up, and you will feel it getting looser. Shoes are also a good indication of hydration. The tighter they are, the more water you need.

FYI: You don't have to drink only water. You can also eat foods with a high water content, such as fruits and vegetables. And finally, research clearly shows that many, many people misinterpret thirst for hunger. The next time you think you are hungry, drink a big glass of water first. I bet you will be surprised.

BUDDY UP

There is strength in numbers. A workout partner provides accountability, which is the key to making any new plan work. If you don't feel like working out, you know in the back of your mind that you are going to let your partner down. That motivates you to crawl out of bed and meet up for the workout. Or if you call and say, "I don't want to," your partner will say,

"Come on, you made me do it last week." A partner will also help with your eating plan. This is especially helpful when you are going to a dinner, party, or event and need to have someone give you strength when the double chocolate fudge cake is served!

HIT THE SCALE

While changes in your body composition will be more apparent in your clothes, the scale still gives you important information regarding the success of your plan. Research from Brown University has shown that the more people weigh themselves, the more they succeed at weight loss. Consider checking your weight two, three, four, or five times a week, but always on the same scale, at the same time. Don't get crazy if you see it fluctuate. Water balance is going to shift, especially for women during ovulation and their monthly cycle or if you have had a high-sodium meal or have recently been on a plane.

In addition to the scale, the best gauge for your body composition shift is your jeans. I tell my clients all the time, "Jeans don't lie," and you should make it a habit to wear them once a week, most likely on Saturday or Sunday. I urge you to wear them on the weekend, because most people tend to eat more on those two days, and the jeans will remind you to be careful.

DOCUMENT

Keeping a food diary and an exercise log is essential to your success. The food diary provides two important functions. One, it allows you to see the numbers to understand what you are eating. Two, it provides you with a tool to self-police. When you are walking through the grocery store and see a plate of smoked sausage samples, or when you pass by the kitchen in the office and see a plate of cookies, reach out and think, *Do I, don't I, do I, don't I? Oh, forget it. I'm not even hungry*. That will be important for keeping your calories down.

I also urge all parents to stop finishing off their kids' food. I know I have done it in the past. You really don't need those leftover fries, chicken tenders, or pizza crusts. You are just popping them in out of habit. Ditto with finishing their cookies. Don't do it.

The exercise log is essential as you apply progression. You think you will "keep it all in your head," but you won't. The more you document, the faster you will progress, because you will look at what you did the last time and push yourself to beat that tension, weight, or rep. I have also frequently used the exercise log as a motivational tool. I will put it right in front of my clients and say, "Can you believe you used to do your back row with the green Xertube and you are all the way up to blue?" They always smile, nod their heads, and put that much more effort into their next set.

I have provided you with sample exercise logs and food diaries in Appendix C.

I also want you to revisit the answers to your questions on page 42 in Chapter 6. On a weekly basis, look at what you originally wrote and how your answers are changing as you succeed with this plan. It will provide you with even more encouragement as you get closer and closer to your ultimate goal.

BE A ROLE MODEL

At this time in our country, the obesity epidemic appears to have taken on a life of its own. According to the American Diabetes Association, "Our nation is experiencing a deterioration of healthy lifestyles of unprecedented proportions that will make future generations sicker." Our children may be the first generation to have shorter life spans than their parents. Compound that with the fact that physical education is being eliminated or phased out of many schools, and realize that many kids practically don't have a chance.

Plus, I'm sure many of your adult friends, family members, and coworkers are in the same place that you are in right now. They, too, are so frustrated from all the attempts at weight loss and have been so burned by bad advice that they just can't muster the energy to give it one more try. A part of me doesn't blame them.

But you can show them the way. You can succeed where so many have failed in the past, because this time you have the right advice and are in the right psychological mind-set to make it happen. Once again, I especially want you to do this for any children or teenagers you see struggling with weight. The number of obese children is rising so rapidly, and very young children are developing medical conditions that used to be found only among much older adults—such as high cholesterol and heart disease, in addition to type 2 diabetes. I don't care whether they are your children, nephews, nieces, or children of your friends and coworkers, kids today need positive role models when it comes to living a healthier lifestyle. Can you even imagine what it must be like to be an overweight teenager in our looks-obsessed, celebrity-driven world these days? I don't believe in preaching or forcing anyone to adopt a healthier eating plan or to exercise. I believe in showing them, by doing it yourself. Prove to them that weight loss and a healthier lifestyle are possible and are within their reach.

And make it fun, don't make it look like work.

That's what I do with my children. Given my profession, I am hypersensitive with how I present healthy eating options and exercise to my kids, as I do not want it to become an issue. My ten-year-old daughter, Olivia, is a big gymnast. So I have told her that her body needs certain foods such as fruits, vegetables, whole grains, and protein, since she is asking it to do so much during practice and competition. She buys in. My son loves wall climbing. It's a great workout, and he takes such pride in making it up to the top as fast as he can. I feel it is a huge confidence builder for him, especially given his sister's success in gymnastics. Yes, his goal in life is to live on chicken tenders and fries, but I am frequently successful in getting many other, healthier options on his plate and into his mouth. Both of my kids love their activities. They were introduced to everything—tennis, dance, soccer, you name it—and they decided what was right for them. I never forced them. You need to help your kids (or children you know who may need some advice in this area) find activities they enjoy.

MINIMIZE STRESS

I know this is easier said than done, but stress has many physical and psychological implications. From a physical standpoint, stress is responsible for sending the hormone cortisol into your bloodstream, and if you recall, cortisol levels increase during high-intensity cardio exercise. Cortisol is frequently maligned in the press, but the truth is, cortisol has been very important to our existence for decades, if not centuries. In the past, when people were in the jungle and were being chased by a wild animal, high cortisol levels enabled them to survive. The surge in cortisol brought energy to their muscles by increasing their heart rate, blood pressure, and breathing so they could run faster. Cortisol also brought a burst of immunity so they could live longer, and it lowered sensitivity to pain. During the cortisol surge, other functions in the body are ignored, such as digestion, sex drive, and even the immune system (I have frequently observed that chronically stressed individuals are sick all the time), so that all energy can be devoted to the stressful situation, which, in the case of our long-ago ancestors, was being chased by a wild animal.

The same thing happens to your body when you are stressed. You get the stress response when needed, but then return to normal, pre-stress levels. Unfortunately, our lives today are so filled with stress that our levels of cortisol stay elevated all the time, because we repeatedly tell the body we are being chased by a wild animal. Then the slightest bit of additional stress (now two wild animals are charging at you) will send cortisol levels skyrocketing. The damaging effects of consistent high cortisol levels include:

- **suppressed thyroid function.** The thyroid produces hormones that regulate metabolism and the function of many other systems of the body. A suppressed thyroid lowers your metabolism.

- **blood sugar imbalances.** Obviously a disaster for those who have issues with blood sugar.

- **decrease in both muscle tissue and bone density.** Isn't this whole book about maintaining and increasing your lean muscle tissue? Cortisol is catabolic, or muscle-depleting. And bone density is essential as we age.

- **high blood pressure.** Once again, a component of allostatic load, which determines how quickly the body ages. And for years we have known that high blood pressure increases the risk of heart disease.

- **suppressed immunity.** The more frequently you get sick, the more excuses you have to stop exercising and turn to comfort food.

- **increased abdominal fat.** Again, this raises your risk of heart disease and diabetes and speeds up the aging process, as waist-to-hip ratio is a component of allostatic load.

To achieve the best results with *The Cardio-Free Diet*, you clearly need to minimize stress.

So just to revisit these seven rules:

1. Sleep—Your hormones (and hips) will thank you.

2. Drink water—You will look *and* feel so much better.

3. Partner up—There is strength in numbers.

4. Weigh in—Don't be afraid to get the data, because you will like what you see.

5. Write it down—It will keep you honest and guarantee effective exercise progression.

6. Set an example—Inspire others with your success.

7. Relax—Take ten slow, deep breaths when you find yourself getting agitated, and please, stop all the damaging cardio.

If you work on these seven rules and strictly follow my eating and exercise plans, your results will be amazing. In exactly eight weeks, you will see your body weight dramatically go down, feel your body's composition significantly change, and experience a surge in your energy levels.

And you never, ever have to step on a treadmill again.

Preventing Diabetes with the Cardio-Free Diet

According to the Centers for Disease Control and Prevention, the average American woman born in 2000 has a 38.5 percent risk of developing diabetes, which will cut her life span by 14.3 years if she is diagnosed by age forty and will reduce the overall quality of her life by 18.6 years. For men born in 2000, that risk is 32.8 percent, and diabetes will shorten his life by 11.6 years if he is diagnosed by age forty and will reduce the quality of his life by 22 years. There is a strong likelihood that children born in the year 2000 (which includes my son, Evan) will be the first generation to have shorter life spans than their parents.

Minority groups fare far worse when it comes to the risk of diabetes, as female and male Hispanics run a 52.5 percent and 51.9 percent risk, respectively, and African-American women and men run a 49 percent and 41.4 percent risk, respectively. White women and men come in lower, at 31.2 percent and 26.7 percent, respectively.

These absolutely frightening statistics are why I felt it was critical to explain how *The Cardio-Free Diet* can reduce your risk of acquiring this debilitating and ultimately deadly disease. It is estimated that 18.2 million Americans already have diabetes. That number has doubled over the past decade and will probably continue to increase at a catastrophic rate. An addition 41 million people are what is considered "prediabetic," which indicates that their fasting blood sugar levels are above normal (anything between eighty and one hundred milligrams per deciliter is considered normal), but not over 126, which is the threshold at which one is considered diabetic. And if you can believe it, up to one-third of all people with diabetes don't even know that they have it.

Diabetes occurs when you have elevated sugar levels traveling around in your bloodstream. There are two classifications of diabetes, type 1 and type 2. Type 1, which used to be called juvenile diabetes, is caused by the death of insulin-producing cells in the pancreas. When we eat, food is converted to glucose, or sugar, so that our cells can use it as fuel. For fuel to enter a cell, insulin must be present. Think of insulin as the drawbridge to entering the castle. When the drawbridge is lowered (insulin is present), glucose can enter the cell (castle). When the drawbridge is up (insulin is not present), then the sugar just runs amuck within the body and does significant damage. With type 1 diabetes, the pancreas just stops making insulin altogether, and the individual is forced to rely on injectable insulin in order to survive and lower his or her sugar levels. Type 1 diabetes is not within your control, as it is hereditary.

With type 2 diabetes, which accounts for 90 to 95 percent of all cases, cells gradually become resistant to insulin over time, as a result of poor diet, lack of exercise, and excess body weight. The glucose comes knocking, but even with the presence of insulin (the drawbridge is down), your cell (the castle) does not allow it to enter as it did in the past, which is referred to as islet cell exhaustion. Therefore, the pancreas furiously pumps out more insulin to eliminate the extra sugar. Finally the pancreas just can't keep up to compensate for the extra sugar, and the cells all but cease even trying to accept the sugar. The pancreas may cease functioning altogether, which causes the person to become insulin-dependent. This occurs either because you are consuming too many foods that rapidly turn to sugar, which are known as high-glycemic foods (generally refined, high-carbohydrate foods), or because you may just have too many cells to service with insulin because of the size of your body.

Researchers at the University of Texas and Yale University are studying how fatty acids floating around in our bloodstream may promote insulin resistance. It makes sense when you consider that most overweight people consume a disproportionate amount of fats and that 85 to 90 percent of all type 2 diabetics are overweight.

Frequently, high sugar levels in your body are compared to rust on a car. Once it starts, it just continues to damage many parts of your vehicle. The same occurs with elevated sugar levels, as the sugar begins to accumulate within the body and attach to places—such as blood vessels, kidneys, and nerves—where it doesn't belong. This can cause heart attack, cancer, stroke, kidney failure, blindness, amputations, nerve damage, impotence, and early death, to name a few. If you recall, blood sugar was one of the components of allostatic load and will therefore also accelerate the aging process.

The Cardio-Free Diet provides a comprehensive plan for minimizing the risk of type 2 diabetes, as it:

1. Reduces your body weight. Weight loss is essential to minimize the risks of diabetes, and research proves that even a modest weight loss of only 5 to 10 percent of total body weight, given that you are already overweight, will reduce blood sugar levels.

2. Increases your lean muscle tissue and reduces your body fat. Similar to weight loss, aerobic conditioning was all that was recommended for diabetics in the past to lower their blood sugar. Now researchers find that weight training alone will help increase glucose uptake by the muscles and help the body to store glucose, or sugar, properly. As you learned in Chapter 10, muscles require that glucose be replenished after strength training in order to rebuild. Anything that helps pull glucose out of the bloodstream is a huge benefit to diabetics. In addition, the increase in your metabolism as a result of the weight training will help insulin function more efficiently.

Very important research recently reported from Michael Goran, PhD, professor of preventative medicine at the Keck School of Medicine at the University of Southern California, showed that overweight Latino boys who performed strength training twice a week for sixteen weeks significantly reduced their risk of insulin resistance. Goran and the other researchers hypothesized that the teens would stick with the strength training more than aerobic exercise because it is less taxing and provides more immediate, recognizable results, which are attributable to the body composition changes attained only through strength training.

The researchers specifically used Latino teens, as more than half of all Latino children born in the year 2000 are expected to suffer from this disease. It is important to note that the researchers kept pushing the participants to continue to use higher resistance and fewer repetitions as the participants increased their strength and lean muscle tissue. This is exactly what I urge you to do as you perform the Cardio-Free Exercise Program.

3. Focuses on high-fiber foods. In Chapter 11 I took you through the Cardio-Free Eating Plan, which places a very high emphasis on whole grain foods, such as brown rice, whole grain cereal, oatmeal, and whole wheat bread. According to a study reported in the *American Journal of Clinical Nutrition*, the high fiber content of whole grains slows down what is called gastric emptying, or the release of glucose into the bloodstream. If the sugar takes longer to be released into the bloodstream, then insulin will not be required to work as hard to clear a way for the sugar to enter the cells. This will also help you feel full for a longer period of time. Whole grains have been shown to have more magnesium, and that also has been shown to improve the insulin response.

4. Recommends fruit. One study asked diabetic patients to consume an apple thirty minutes before breakfast, lunch, and dinner. The result? These patients significantly reduced their blood sugar. The researchers felt that the high fiber content in the apples and the fact-that they helped participants feel full led to lower total caloric consumption and subsequently lower blood sugar levels.

5. Significantly reduces juice and other liquid calorie consumption. As you have seen in the eating plan, juice, sports drinks, soda, and high-calorie coffee and tea drinks should be drastically reduced for those with diabetes and those who wish to lose weight.

6. Allows you to consume wine. In Phase II of the eating plan, you are allowed one glass of wine a day. This is beneficial to those with elevated blood sugar levels. Australian researchers found that consuming one and a half glasses of wine *after* a meal brings insulin levels back to pre-meal levels. Just skip the supersweet dessert wines. Plus, it is well documented that a glass of wine has heart-health benefits, and diabetics are at a significantly greater risk of heart disease.

7. Emphasizes nuts. Harvard researchers reported that women who consume an ounce of nuts or peanut butter five times a week reduced their risk of type 2 diabetes by approximately 21 percent (this has been done for you in the Cardio-Free Eating Plan). They stated that nuts contain a lot of the good fats—mono- or polyunsaturated—which help both cholesterol levels and insulin sensitivity. Nuts are very high in fiber, similar to whole wheat products and fruit, and also contain vitamins, minerals, and plant protein. It is important, however, to keep the portion of nuts small, as the calories add up quickly.

8. Insists that you eat breakfast. An eight-year Harvard study showed that people who ate breakfast were half as likely to develop insulin resistance.

9. Promotes dairy products. The *Journal of the American Medical Association* found that those who consume the most dairy products each week were 72 percent less likely to develop insulin sensitivity. You have also learned that dairy is key to promoting weight loss.

10. Urges you to sleep. Sleep, as you learned in Chapter 13, is essential to maintaining a lower body weight and reducing the risk of type 2 diabetes. Researchers have shown that those who sleep less than six and a half hours a night have a 40 percent lower insulin sensitivity than those who sleep closer to eight.

In conclusion, *The Cardio-Free Diet* can greatly benefit those who are diabetic, prediabetic, or know (because of family history, current eating habits, or present body weight) that they are at risk. The sooner you can minimize the damage of high sugar levels in your bloodstream, the better off you will be.

APPENDIX B

Shopping Lists

Here are eight shopping lists that correspond to the eight-week eating plan. In the shopping list for week 1, I have included certain products that will be used for the entire eight-week period. If you already have any of these products, just delete them from the list.

I recommend that you buy some of the fruits and vegetables at a salad bar in the grocery store. That way, you buy only what you need, which will minimize the chance of overeating, and it will be convenient.

Week 1 Shopping List

FRUITS/VEGETABLES	QUANTITY
Kiwi	1
Orange	1
Pears	2
Lime	1
Strawberries	3 cups
Cranberries	¾ cup
Blueberries	2 cups
Raspberries	1 cup
Apples	3
Tomatoes	5
Cherry tomatoes	10
Celery	1 stalk
Green peppers	6
Red pepper	1

Broccoli (florets)	8 cups
Mushrooms	3 cups
Carrots	2 cups
Asparagus spears	16
Cucumber	1
Zucchini	3
Yellow squash	1
Onion	1
Parsley	¾ cup
Garlic	2 cloves
Spinach	1 bag
Mixed greens	3 bags
Romaine lettuce	2 leaves

*MEN ADD:

Pineapple	2 cups
Banana	1
Apple	1
Honeydew	1½ cups
Celery	1 stalk
Raisins	⅓ cup

DAIRY	**QUANTITY**
Eggs	16
Feta cheese	1 4-ounce container

String cheese	1 package of 8
2% cottage cheese	2 16-ounce containers
100-calorie low-fat yogurt	5 6-ounce containers
Nonfat or low-fat banana yogurt	1 6-ounce container
Low-fat vanilla yogurt	1 6-ounce container
1% milk	1 pint
Shredded low-fat cheddar cheese	1 bag
Laughing Cow Light Garlic & Herb cheese	1 wedge

*MEN ADD:

Egg	1
2% cottage cheese	1 24-ounce container

MEAT/FISH	QUANTITY
Boneless, skinless chicken breast	19 ounces
Low-fat (99% fat free, if possible) ground turkey	9 ounces
Swordfish	6 ounces
Salmon	6 ounces
Whitefish fillet	5 ounces
Low-fat sliced turkey	1 small package
Tuna steak	5 ounces

FROZEN	QUANTITY
Shrimp	1 2-pound bag

*MEN ADD:

Edamame	½ cup

GROCERIES	QUANTITY
Fat-free cooking spray	1 can
Balsamic vinegar	1 bottle
Raspberry vinegar	1 bottle
Lemon juice	1 bottle
Tomato juice	1 small can
Salt	1 shaker
Black pepper	1 shaker
Chili powder	1 shaker
Garlic powder	1 shaker
Ketchup	1 bottle
Yellow mustard	1 bottle
Chickpeas	¼ cup
Fat-free ranch dressing	1 bottle
Canned kidney beans	1 can
Spicy mustard	1 bottle
Almonds	1 16-ounce can
Roasted peanuts	1 16-ounce can
Peanut butter	1 jar
Corn tortillas	1 package

Wheaties	1 box
Whole wheat bread	1 loaf
Reduced-Fat Wheat Thins	1 box
Reduced-Fat Triscuits	1 box
Plain instant oatmeal	1 box with individual packages
Crushed tomatoes	4 ounces
Dried basil	1 jar
Dried oregano	1 jar

*MEN ADD:

| Raisins | 1 box |

Week 2 Shopping List

FRUITS/VEGETABLES	QUANTITY
Mandarin oranges	2
Honeydew	1
Apples	3
Nectarines	3
Apricots	2
Pineapple	1
Grapefruit	1
Strawberries	3½ cups
Blueberries	2 cups
Raspberries	½ cup
Seedless grapes	1 1-pound bag
Banana	1
Tomatoes	4
Roma tomatoes	2
Cherry tomatoes	20
Green peppers	6
Yellow peppers	1
Cucumbers	2
Zucchini	2
Yellow squash	1
Baby carrots	1 bag

Mushrooms	2 cups
Onion	1
Broccoli (florets)	9 cups
Artichoke hearts	½ cup
Green beans	2 cups
Romaine lettuce	1 bag
Sprouts	1 cup
Garlic	2 cloves
Parsley leaves	2 sprigs
Mixed greens	3 bags
Carrots	3 cups

*MEN ADD:

Kiwis	2
Banana	1
Tomato	1

DAIRY	**QUANTITY**
Eggs	8
2% cottage cheese	2 16-ounce containers
100-calorie low-fat yogurt	4 6-ounce containers
Low-fat vanilla yogurt	2 6-ounce containers
Low-fat American cheese slices	1 small package
1% milk	1 pint

*MEN ADD:

Egg	1
String cheese	1 package of 8
2% cottage cheese	1 24-ounce container

MEAT/FISH	QUANTITY
White meat lean roast turkey	3 ounces
Boneless, skinless chicken breast	16 ounces
Low-fat turkey breast slices	1 small package
Ground lean turkey	4 ounces
Lean pork chops	4 ounces
Haddock fillet	6 ounces
Cod fillet	4 ounces

FROZEN	QUANTITY
*MEN:	
Edamame	½ cup

GROCERIES	QUANTITY
Canned light tuna in water	3 ounces
Dry white wine	1 bottle
Thyme	1 jar
Rosemary	1 jar

Cinnamon	1 jar
Ginger	1 jar
Tomato paste	1 can
Marinara sauce	1 jar
Dried cranberries	1 bag
Cashew nuts	1 16-ounce can
Low-fat cream of mushroom soup	1 can
Graham crackers	1 box
All-fruit spread	1 jar
Whole wheat tortilla	1
Dijon mustard	1 jar

Week 3 Shopping List

FRUITS/VEGETABLES	QUANTITY
Oranges	2
Mandarin oranges	2
Apples	4
Lime	1
Pineapple	1
Lemon	1
Strawberries	6 cups
Blueberries	1 cup
Raspberries	3½ cups
Banana	1
Peach	1
Mango	1
Tomatoes	6
Cherry tomatoes	10
Celery	4 stalks
Broccoli (florets)	2 cups
Baby carrots	1 bag
Green beans	4 cups
Green onions	1
Green peppers	3
Red onion	1
Red cabbage	½ cup
Fresh ginger	1 teaspoon

Red pepper	1
Zucchini	2
Onion	1
Garlic	1 clove
Cucumbers	3
Asparagus spears	12
Mushrooms	1 cup
Spinach leaves	3 bags
Carrots	2 cups

*MEN ADD:

Apples	2
Strawberries	½ cup
Kiwis	2
Pineapple	1
Blueberries	3 cups
Celery	1 stalk

DAIRY	QUANTITY
Eggs	8
2% cottage cheese	1 24-ounce container
String cheese	1 package of 8
Feta cheese	1 4-ounce container
100-calorie low-fat yogurt	5 6-ounce containers

| Low-fat banana yogurt | 1 6-ounce container |
| 1% milk | 1 pint |

*MEN ADD:

| 2% cottage cheese | 1 16-ounce container |

MEAT/FISH	QUANTITY
Boneless, skinless chicken breast	22 ounces
Low-fat sliced turkey	1 small package
Tuna steak	6 ounces

FROZEN	QUANTITY
Veggie burgers	1 box

GROCERIES	QUANTITY
Apricot preserves	1 jar
Fat-free mayonnaise	1 jar
Nutmeg	1 jar
Cider vinegar	1 container
Salsa	1 container
Curry powder	1 shaker
Sugar	1 small package
Soy sauce	1 small bottle
Cilantro	1 jar

Canned tuna in water	2 6-ounce cans
MultiGrain Cheerios	1 small box
Wild rice	1 box
Whole wheat bread	1 loaf
Corn tortillas	1 package
Pickle spears	1 jar

Week 4 Shopping List

FRUITS/VEGETABLES	QUANTITY
Kiwis	2
Apples	4
Pear	1
Peach	1
Nectarines	2
Pineapple	1
Lemon	1
Strawberries	3 cups
Blueberries	3½ cups
Green peppers	3
Red pepper	1
Green beans	2 cups
Celery	6 stalks
Carrots	4¼ cups
Broccoli (florets)	10 cups
Bean sprouts	1 cup
Mushrooms	1 cup
Tomatoes	2
Zucchini	5
Cucumber	1
Yellow squash	2
Potato	1

Black olives	4
Fresh basil	2 tablespoons
Mixed greens 2 bags	2 bags
Romaine lettuce	4 leaves
Spinach leaves	1 bag

*MEN ADD:

Apple	1
Kiwis	2
Strawberries	½ cup
Blueberries	1 cup
Celery	3 stalks

DAIRY	QUANTITY
Eggs	5
2% cottage cheese	2 24-ounce containers
Low-fat sliced American cheese	1 small package
Low-fat mozzarella cheese	1 package
1% milk	1 pint
Shredded low-fat cheddar cheese	1 ounce
100-calorie low-fat yogurt	3 6-ounce containers

*MEN ADD:

Egg	1
2% cottage cheese	1 16-ounce container

MEAT/FISH	QUANTITY
Boneless, skinless chicken breast	17 ounces
Low-fat turkey bacon	1 small package
Low-fat turkey slices	1 small package
Sara Lee honey ham	1 small package
Low-fat sliced chicken	1 small package
Flounder fillet	7 ounces
Poached salmon fillet	6 ounces
Halibut	4 ounces

GROCERIES	QUANTITY
Cumin	1 jar
Honey mustard	1 bottle
Canned diced tomatoes	1 can
Canned kidney beans	1 can
Special K	1 box
Brown rice	1 box
Fat-free flour tortilla	1 package
Raisin Bran	1 box
Tomato juice	4 tablespoons

Week 5 Shopping List

FRUITS/VEGETABLES	QUANTITY
Kiwi	1
Orange	1
Pears	2
Lime	1
Strawberries	3½ cups
Cranberries	1 cup
Blueberries	2 cups
Raspberries	1 cup
Apples	4
Tomatoes	6
Cherry tomatoes	10
Celery	1 stalk
Green peppers	7
Red peppers	2
Broccoli (florets)	11 cups
Mushrooms	3½ cups
Carrots	2½ cups
Asparagus spears	20
Cucumber	1
Zucchini	4
Yellow squash	1

Onion	1
Garlic	2 cloves
Parsley	¾ cup
Spinach	1 bag
Mixed greens	4 bags

*MEN ADD:

Pineapple	1
Banana	1
Apple	1
Honeydew	1½ cups
Celery	1 stalk

DAIRY	**QUANTITY**
Eggs	17
Shredded low-fat cheddar cheese	1 package
Feta cheese	1 4-ounce container
String cheese	1 package of 8
2% cottage cheese	2 16-ounce containers
100-calorie low-fat yogurt	5 6-ounce containers
Nonfat or 1% banana yogurt	1 6-ounce container
Low-fat vanilla yogurt	1 6-ounce container
1% milk	1 pint
Laughing Cow Light Garlic & Herb cheese	3 wedges

*MEN ADD:

Egg	1
Laughing Cow Light Garlic & Herb cheese	3 wedges
2% cottage cheese	1 24-ounce container

MEAT/FISH	QUANTITY
Boneless, skinless chicken breast	24 ounces
Low-fat ground turkey	11 ounces
Swordfish	7 ounces
Salmon	7 ounces
Whitefish fillet	6 ounces
Low-fat sliced turkey	1 small package
Tuna steak	6 ounces

FROZEN	QUANTITY
Shrimp	1 2-pound bag

*MEN ADD:

Edamame	½ cup

GROCERIES	QUANTITY
Chickpeas	¼ cup
Canned kidney beans	½ cup
Spicy mustard	1 bottle
Almonds	1 16-ounce can

Roasted peanuts	1 16-ounce can
Corn tortillas	1 package
Whole wheat bread	1 loaf
Plain instant oatmeal	1 box with individual packets

*MEN ADD:

Raisins	1 box

Week 6 Shopping List

FRUITS/VEGETABLES	QUANTITY
Mandarin oranges	2
Honeydew	1
Apples	5
Nectarines	3
Apricots	2
Pineapple	1
Grapefruit	1
Strawberries	3½ cups
Blueberries	2 cups
Raspberries	½ cup
Seedless grapes	1 bag
Banana	1
Tomatoes	4
Roma tomatoes	2
Cherry tomatoes	20
Green peppers	7
Yellow peppers	1
Cucumbers	2
Zucchini	2
Yellow squash	1
Baby carrots	1 bag

Mushrooms	2 cups
Onion	1
Carrots	5 cups
Broccoli	10½ cups
Artichoke hearts	½ cup
Green beans	3 cups
Sprouts	1 cup
Garlic	2 cloves
Parsley leaves	2 sprigs
Mixed greens	3 bags
Romaine lettuce	1 bag
Asparagus spears	8

*MEN ADD:

Kiwis	2
Banana	1
Tomato	1

DAIRY	**QUANTITY**
Eggs	12
2% cottage cheese	2 16-ounce containers
100-calorie low-fat yogurt	4 6-ounce containers
Low-fat vanilla yogurt	2 6-ounce containers
Low-fat American cheese slices	1 small package
1% milk	1 pint

*MEN ADD:

Egg	1
String cheese	1 package of 8
2% cottage cheese	1 24-ounce container

FROZEN

QUANTITY

*MEN:

Edamame	½ cup

MEAT/FISH

QUANTITY

White meat lean roast turkey	2 cups
Boneless, skinless chicken breast	20 ounces
Low-fat turkey breast slices	1 small package
Ground lean turkey	5 ounces
Lean pork chops	6 ounces
Haddock fillet	9 ounces
Cod fillet	6 ounces

GROCERIES

QUANTITY

Canned tuna in water	3 ounces
Tomato paste	1 can
Marinara sauce	1 jar
Cashew nuts	1 16-ounce can
Low-fat cream of mushroom soup	1 can

Week 7 Shopping List

FRUITS/VEGETABLES	QUANTITY
Oranges	2
Mandarin oranges	2
Apples	5
Lime	1
Pineapple	1
Lemon	1
Strawberries	7 cups
Blueberries	1 cup
Raspberries	3½ cups
Banana	1
Peach	1
Mango	1
Tomatoes	6
Cherry tomatoes	10
Celery	4 stalks
Broccoli (florets)	3 cups
Baby carrots	1 bag
Green beans	6½ cups
Green onions	1
Green peppers	3
Fresh ginger	1 teaspoon
Carrots	2½ cups
Red onion	1

Red cabbage	½ cup
Red pepper	1
Zucchini	2
Onion	1
Garlic	1 clove
Cucumbers	4
Asparagus spears	16
Mushrooms	1 cup
Red-tipped lettuce	4 leaves
Green lettuce	2 leaves
Spinach leaves	3 bags

*MEN ADD:

Apples	2
Kiwis	2
Pineapple	1
Strawberries	½ cup
Blueberries	3 cups
Celery	1 stalk

DAIRY	**QUANTITY**
Eggs	12
2% cottage cheese	1 24-ounce container
String cheese	1 package of 8
Feta cheese	1 4-ounce container
100-calorie low-fat yogurt	5 6-ounce containers

Low-fat banana yogurt	1 6-ounce container
1% milk	1 pint

*MEN ADD:

2% cottage cheese	1 12-ounce container

MEAT/FISH	QUANTITY
Boneless, skinless chicken breast	27 ounces
Low-fat sliced turkey	1 package
Tuna steak	7 ounces

GROCERIES	QUANTITY
Apricot preserves	1 jar
Salsa	1 container
Canned light tuna in water	3 6-ounce cans
Whole wheat bread	1 loaf

Week 8 Shopping List

FRUITS/VEGETABLES	QUANTITY
Kiwis	2
Apples	5
Pear	1
Peach	1
Nectarines	2
Pineapple	1
Lemon	1
Strawberries	3 cups
Blueberries	5½ cups
Green peppers	5
Red peppers	2
Green beans	3 cups
Celery	6 stalks
Carrots	6½ cups
Broccoli (florets)	13 cups
Bean sprouts	1 cup
Mushrooms	1 cup
Tomatoes	2
Zucchini	6
Cucumber	1
Yellow squash	3
Potato	1
Black olives	4

Fresh basil	2 tablespoons
Mixed greens	2 bags
Romaine lettuce	4 leaves
Spinach leaves	1 bag

*MEN ADD:

Apple	1
Kiwis	2
Blueberries	1 cup
Strawberries	½ cup
Celery	3 stalks

DAIRY	**QUANTITY**
Eggs	8
2% cottage cheese	2 24-ounce containers
Low-fat mozzarella cheese	1 8-ounce package
1% milk	1 pint
100-calorie low-fat yogurt	3 6-ounce containers

*MEN ADD:

Eggs	1
2% cottage cheese	1 16-ounce container

MEAT/FISH	**QUANTITY**
Boneless, skinless chicken breast	21 ounces
Low-fat turkey bacon	1 small package
Low-fat turkey slices	1 small package

Sara Lee honey ham	1 small package
Low-fat sliced chicken	1 small package
Flounder fillet	9 ounces
Poached salmon fillet	7 ounces
Halibut	6 ounces

GROCERIES	QUANTITY
Canned diced tomatoes	1 can
Canned kidney beans	2 cans
Chickpeas	¼ cup

Exercise Logs and Daily Food Diaries

PROGRAM ONE

EQUIPMENT

Using SPRI Xertube, Door
Attachment, and Lex Loop

Xertube (T)
Door Attachment (D)
Lex Loop (L)

	Exercise	Equipment		1	2	3	4	5	6	7	8
								WEEK			
1	Back Row on Both Legs	T, D	Color								
			Reps								
2	Hip Extension	L	Color								
			Reps								
3	Chest Press (on both legs)	T, D	Color								
			Reps								
4	Lying-Down Hip Abduction	L	Color								
			Reps								
5	Bicep Curl	T	Color								
			Reps								
6	Drop-Step Abduction	L	Color								
			Reps								
7	Tricep Pushdown	T, D	Color								
			Reps								
8	Abdominal Crunch	T, D	Color								
			Reps								
9	Standing Hamstring Curl	L	Color								
			Reps								
10	Rear Deltoid Fly (on both legs)	T, D	Color								
			Reps								
11	Straight-Arms Pushdown (on one leg)	T, D	Color								
			Reps								
12	Plank (Lex Loop around ankles)	L	Color								
			Reps								
13	Standing Hip Abduction	L	Color								
			Reps								
14	Lateral Raise (in lunge position)	T	Color								
			Reps								
15	Lat Pulldown	T, D	Color								
			Reps								
16	Shoulder Press (in squat position)	T	Color								
			Reps								

PROGRAM TWO   EQUIPMENT

Using Free Weights

Single Dumbbell (1)
Both Dumbbells (2)
Body Weight Only (B)

#	Exercise	Equipment		WEEK 1	2	3	4	5	6	7	8
1	One-Arm Row (with opposite arm out to your side)	1	Lbs / Reps								
2	Stationary Lunges	2	Lbs / Reps								
3	Push-up	B	Lbs / Reps								
4	Squat	2	Lbs / Reps								
5	Shoulder Press	2	Lbs / Reps								
6	Dead Lift	2	Lbs / Reps								
7	Bicep Curl	2	Lbs / Reps								
8	Abdominal Bicycle	B	Lbs / Reps								
9	One-Leg Reach	1	Lbs / Reps								
10	Bent-Over Rear Deltoid Fly	2	Lbs / Reps								
11	Back-Stepping Lunges	2	Lbs / Reps								
12	Lying-Down Tricep Extension (while bridging)	2	Lbs / Reps								
13	Side Plank	B	Lbs / Reps								
14	Bridge Pullover	1	Lbs / Reps								
15	Superman	1	Lbs / Reps								
16	Prone Pulldown	2	Lbs / Reps								

DAILY FOOD DIARY

*Phase/Day:*_____

MEAL	FOODS	PORTION SIZE	CALORIES
Breakfast			
Snack #1			
Lunch			
Snack #2			
Dinner			
Snack #3			

TOTAL
CALORIES: